"The breadth of the territory this book most. . . . Her down-to-earth suggesti real people, young and old, as they s an especially valuable handbook for anyone caught in its grip—and for those trying to help them escape it."

—Lisa Alther, author of *Kinflicks* and *Swan Song*

"I'm quite certain Stephanie wrote this book for me. It's an absolute lifeline for anyone with anxiety."

—Dr. Jodi Richardson, speaker, author, and host of *Well, hello anxiety* podcast

"With a deep understanding of not just the psychological but biological aspects, Stephanie Dowrick shares real-life, real-world tools and how to create a self-therapy healing practice that works."

—Kris Ferraro, international energy healer, speaker, and author of *Your Difference Is Your Strength*

"Stephanie Dowrick's writing is like sunshine for the growth of our 'wise self.' Her words nurture the seeds of kindness, creativity, generosity, aliveness, and presence that lie within us all. Stephanie's words and insights have enriched my life with wisdom, hope, and courage."

—Marie Bismark, professor and consultant psychiatrist

Your name is not Anxious

A very personal guide to putting anxiety in its place

STEPHANIE DOWRICK

ST. MARTIN'S
ESSENTIALS
NEW YORK

First published in the United States by St. Martin's Essentials, an imprint of St. Martin's Publishing Group

YOUR NAME IS NOT ANXIOUS. Copyright © 2024 by Stephanie Dowrick. All rights reserved. Printed in the United States of America. For information, address St. Martin's Publishing Group, 120 Broadway, New York, NY 10271.

www.stmartins.com

The Library of Congress Cataloging-in-Publication Data is available upon request.

ISBN 978-1-250-35517-1 (trade paperback)
ISBN 978-1-250-35518-8 (ebook)

Our books may be purchased in bulk for promotional, educational, or business use. Please contact your local bookseller or the Macmillan Corporate and Premium Sales Department at 1-800-221-7945, extension 5442, or by email at MacmillanSpecialMarkets@macmillan.com.

Originally published in Australia by Allen & Unwin
First published in the United States by St. Martin's Essentials
First U.S. Edition: 2025

For my family, and for yours

Contents

Part Three **Putting anxiety in its place**

The world has never been more crazy . . .
[but] how amazing is it for this very short time to be alive.
BILL BRYSON

The most common way people give up their power
is by thinking they don't have any.
ALICE WALKER

If life were predictable, it would cease to be life.
RUPI KAUR

Note to readers

Both anxiety and stress disempower us, sometimes gravely, but they certainly affect every aspect of our lives, including our most fundamental sense of self.

It's my personal and clinical knowledge of how outrageously disempowering anxiety can be that inspired me to write this book—and to write it in the way that I have. *I wanted to return power to you.* Discovering that *anxiety is the most treatable of mood disruptions* made me even more determined to make such re-empowerment effective. Particularly to regain the precious inner sense of choice and well-being that anxiety disrupts or takes away.

We know that knowledge is power. When it comes to the multiple ways that anxiety affects (and infects) our lives, that saying is neon-lit. *Anxiety is treatable because so much is now known about its effects on mind (yes), body (yes, yes), and how we think about and judge or encourage ourselves (spirit).* Yet even with the best therapy or counseling intentions, those vital connections, plus the neurobiological interconnections between stress and anxiety, are often not emphasized strongly enough to achieve lasting change.

This is a book of practical strategies to share that knowledge—and to re-empower. It is support close at hand that offers *informed* guidance and, in this instance, many inspiring stories (and some memoir) to bring that guidance to life. Here, the stories have layers of benefit. *Storytelling is the default position of the brain.* It is our primary means to explore and better understand life. Yet, in shifting the way that our emotions and moods work for or against us, we need strategies even more than the stories that illustrate them. We need them fast. We need them to be strong, embracing, and strengthening.

I'm aware that the people suffering most from anxiety already likely feel emotionally flooded. Taking in lots of information is horribly hard when you are under siege. My way around this was to create short chapters with highly descriptive titles, and to repeat key ideas and concepts throughout the book. This means that wherever you dive in you will find something that supports you *right now* through whatever else is going on.

**You don't have to read this book from
beginning to end to "get it."
You can meet the most useful, transformative
ideas expressed across a variety of circumstances,
and in many different ways.**

What I am writing about here—anxiety—is intensely personal. Positive inner shifts will come when you have that moment of personal recognition. That's when an idea, an insight, new research, or a shared inspiration jumps from my page into your life. May there be many such moments for you here in these pages. May they make the difference you are seeking.

Making this book your own

*The way you look at things is the most
powerful force in shaping your life.*

JOHN O'DONOHUE

"She's always anxious, haven't you noticed?"

"I'm a trained psychologist who has panic attacks."

*"I can't persuade my partner/friend/child/brother to do anything out of the
ordinary. Too much stress they say."*

"You think I'm self-assured! What a joke."

*"I used to like the push that tension and anxiety gave me. But then I found
I was facing every moment as though it was a test."*

"Until I had my first baby, I was fine. Since then, I see danger everywhere."

*"What I worry most about is all too real. But I can't turn it off or tone it
down."*

**Shifting your relationship with anxiety, if it is uncomfortable
or limiting, shifts the way you see yourself. It also shifts the
way you see and interact with other people. Understanding**

1

yourself and what's happening in your mind is never about your mind only. It's never about your body and mind only.

It's about your stance in the world.

Your name is not Anxious comes to you as a book to use, not just read. And to use in your own way. The core idea here can be life-changing: *You are more than your anxiety, however controlling it may currently be.* You are also much more than any emotions or thoughts that seem to be defeating you. But to bring that more complete, truer picture of yourself to life, it needs to become real to you.

This is not a book only "about" anxiety. There are plenty of those. It is first and foremost a book about you, and about how anxiety is *limiting the way you see yourself.*

I came to this writing after two hard years of observing in a beloved family member how dangerous anxiety can be when it is poorly understood and inadequately treated, *even when that treatment is "evidence-based" and comes with the best of intentions.* It was not only the loss of peace of mind that I witnessed, but it was also a serious loss of pleasure in living, joy in the small "ordinary" moments of existence, easy laughter, a sense of the ridiculous, and confidence in her own self-worth.

In some desperation, I asked myself repeatedly what insights would make a difference and whether a more generous view might soften the painful reactions and behaviors that trip someone up repeatedly, despite their courage and intelligence.

I reluctantly recognized, too, that all the reassurances in the world can't give someone else a more compassionate reality. It has to be sought. And found—not through any magic, but through undoing harmful attitudes, and welcoming truer, kinder interpretations and perspectives.

Persistent anxiety often follows depression, or vice versa. How could it not? The roots of anxiety run deep.

The potent mix of anxiety and depression has been my personal reality also, even though my own most intense periods of anxiety haven't taken me to the brink in the way my family member has endured. At the worst moments, she would say, anguished, "No one understands, no one understands."

Will you find some understanding here? I more than hope so. And *self*-understanding above everything. This changes the power of the Inner Critic, the undermining whispers that tell you everything is sure to be wrong, and nothing will ever be quite right. Those whisperings are powerful, and never empowering. They are fed by stress, panic, exhaustion, anxiety—and the physiological effects that rush through you. What can change? What you tell yourself, most of all. What you most identify with. What comes to feel dominant. Or less so. And the effect this has on your entire sense of being.

Storytelling is the default position of the brain. A limited view of yourself is corrosive. It causes increasing damage to your inner world, even if you can put on a bright face, or outwork any competitor. Piecemeal change to undermining thoughts is always possible. Yet, *without a fundamental shift in* how you see yourself, *you remain vulnerable.* You remain especially vulnerable to your need for other people to be reassuring or praising you before you can feel "real."

Insight, it must be emphasized, is never enough. It is the yin without the yang. A *"good idea" needs to land in the day-to-day reality of your existence.* It needs to motivate a change in behavior. The parallel would be to sit with a beatific smile on your face while you are on your meditation cushion thinking lovely thoughts but then get up and are furious because someone has done one of a thousand things that disrupt your fixed agenda. The cushion experience may bring plenty of insight. All is lost, as if it had never been, if changed action doesn't reflect your nobler thoughts!

Getting that bigger sense of yourself starts with at least a partial willingness to feel in your bones and your soul, "Anxiety is not all of who I am. Yes, it can affect my whole body and especially my instincts and feelings. It can confuse me. It can devastate me. Nonetheless, *I* am not anxiety and *anxiety* is not what I am."

This shift changes how you see yourself and your ability to connect and cope. It also changes the way you will think about and experiment with creative change in the actions and behaviors that bring your best intentions to life.

When anxiety seems to be running the show, what's needed is a passionate, life-affirming response. Using self-therapy that connects insight and effective action puts you at the center of change. The gifts self-therapy brings are three-fold: 1) needed insight into how your life could be calmer and (much) more pleasurable; 2) a renewal of *self-trust* that you can be in charge of any change; 3) *presence of mind to choose your responses, rather than being driven by habitual reactions.*

Impossible? In one great gulp, maybe yes. Through lived daily experiences—and a far more self-supporting way of thinking about them—it makes a lot of sense.

The chapter headings here are self-explanatory. Dive in wherever a heading tells you, "This is for me." Trust your instincts for positive change. Trust, too, that the way the book is written, core ideas appear and reappear, just as they will in your own mind.

When you do feel fragile or extra distressed, you will want something to hold on to in those moments. I have written some chapters (part two) to use in exactly that way.

It was only through observing and caring for our family member that I fully realized how dangerous high levels of anxiety or all-consuming dread can be. Also, that this is more than a mental health issue: not just the whole self needs understanding, *it is a whole-body response and care that offers essential benefits.*

Everything I thought I knew had to be revised.

All the emergency measures offered here involve the body and ways to acknowledge and soothe the messages coming from the brain (especially the amygdala and hippocampus) that set up whole-body stress responses and rising levels of stress hormones (including cortisol). These are magnificent lifesaving responses in an emergency. They are far less so when stress hormone levels are stuck on "high."

(The amygdala is where "fear memories" are stored, some of which may be triggered by a new situation. More positively, the amygdala is also involved in rewards. Nothing in our whole-body systems works independently—how could it?)

Learning and practicing ways to soothe yourself is basic self-care—and makes so much more sense once you know what involuntary physiological and neurological effects accompany chronic or acute anxiety. Using your body (and breath) to calm your mind is wonderful body-mind cooperation.

When your situation is less urgent and you can manage to soothe yourself so things *feel less urgent*, you can access your "emotional brain" plus your "thinking brain"—the prefrontal cortex and the last area of the brain to develop in you. That's also the last area of the brain to develop in our species, 250 million years after the initial "body brain" or "survival brain" that does such magnificent work for your survival but cannot help you think your way out of difficult or challenging situations.

My training has been psychological and spiritual, which brings understanding and meaning. This is profound. And as we look for a whole-self, whole-body picture, it is quite obviously limited! Chronic or acute anxiety impacts your "moods" and outlook—and your whole body, along with your fundamental sense of self and self-trust. This affects your interactions with other people, including (or especially) those you care about most.

Know, too, that you are inevitably dealing with your own anxiety in a time of unprecedented global stress, chaotic demands, crazy competitiveness, and galloping anxiety in all age groups. Everywhere you look there are gross imbalances of power. We feel that deep inside ourselves. Yet, it's widely expected that you will deal with that external stress, and the anxiety that comes with it, individually. And if that doesn't work, you may be referred to services that will be stretched, necessarily fitting you into a treatment formula that only touches the edge. *But even if you get superb help, no therapist or psychologist can be with you at every moment. Nor should they be.*

My goal is to give you the means to be your own best and best-informed supporter, *affected by anxiety but not diminished by it*.

The insight/action self-therapy offered here will help most, though, when you find yourself in these pages, when you discover what "fits" and *go further with that than I have. No one knows more than you do about your own life—or what you long for. No one knows which stories spun in your own mind enlarge your sense of yourself, or fragment it.* Anxiety, after all, does many things, but it cannot encourage the subtle, creative, self-trusting attitudes you need. It doesn't value curiosity. It doesn't inspire you to be more appreciative, more forgiving, more enchanted with life. Self-valuing like that does more than reduce the pain anxiety brings. It can recharge your entire being.

Last, but definitely not least, what I also offer here—as a creative writer trained in psychotherapy and ministry—is a raft of ways to discover and use your own unique creativity.

Creativity is the asset that will seldom fail you. It is a way of living (and regarding yourself) that lets you see new possibilities, rather than closed exits that might already have failed you. It is also a way of further befriending your mind, particularly if you feel your body-mind has been letting you down.

It lets you discover day by day and experience by experience the continuously unfolding promise of your life. It lets you ask, *"What's needed here?"* Or, *"Is there another way of looking at this?"* Or even, *"How would a really calm, wise person look at this?"*

Simply asking those kinds of questions gets your mind moving. You will discover that any positive shift of perspective brings energy as well as hope.

Creativity means bringing forward a fresh response from your own mind and your invaluable lived experience. It's a prompt toward a less linear or habitual way of thinking about difficulties. This shift lets you live more empathically and generously with others, making it much easier, for example, to see things from someone else's point of view— or to switch your own point of view when that's helpful. It's about finding ways to focus less on what divides and more on what unites. It is the vital prism through which to view your "whole self."

Are you already saying, though, "Me? Creative? Are you kidding?"

> **No one who suffers from anxiety's many forms has a weak imagination. On the contrary, you are likely to have a very strong imagination when it comes to what *might go wrong*. Or even for catastrophic thinking. *This same imaginative power can work for you rather than against you*, opening new possibilities as they are needed, empowering you across every aspect of your existence.**

Part One

You are more than your anxiety

1 | The absolute basics

Anxiety is not "all in the mind." It affects your whole body, and certainly your emotions. Those big responses you are feeling to immediate or potential unsettling or frightening situations happen within your body. They are driven by complex systems outside your immediate control that are doing exactly what they should: alerting you to danger so you can protect yourself. However, when "alerting" becomes too frequent, or semipermanent, this is exhausting and destabilizing. Something needs to be done. *Something can be done.*

1. *Anxiety is treatable.* It is the most treatable of all "mood disorders." This puts power back where it belongs—with you. However good your support, you are the most vital member of your "treating team."

2. Managing stress and *reducing it wherever possible* is your first major step in taking back power—and putting yourself in charge of your moods and emotions. *This is not optional.* Stress and anxiety

are inextricably linked. No one but you can sort your priorities and *put your well-being first*.

3. Anxiety expresses instincts, feelings, and reactions that have a vital place in a healthy psyche. *But anxiety should never dominate.* Nor should it dominate the way you think about yourself.

4. You live in a wondrous physical world, and an often insanely stressful, hectic, and competitive one. *Anxiety is a rational response to a world like ours.* But you can reduce its sting.

5. *A whole-self perspective embraces all that you are. Habits of thinking and feeling are only that—habits. Some are supporting you. Some are not.* You are always more than your thoughts and feelings, however persuasive they may be.

6. When you are acutely anxious, *calm your body first.* When you are less anxious, you can use strategies and insights that radically broaden your choices.

7. *Self-therapy brings invaluable insights from all your experiences. It gives back* the power and choices that anxiety has taken away. If you have professional help, self-therapy can augment it, supporting you 24/7.

8. *Insight and action are self-therapy essentials.* Without action, insight fizzles into nothing (no change). Without insight, you will lack the motivation to create meaningful change—and benefit from it.

9. *Pay close attention to where you give your time and attention.* Reduce what lowers your spirits and elevates your stress levels. Living with Zen equanimity is not the goal. Feeling fully alive is.

10. *Befriend your mind*—especially if you feel that your mind (along with your brain) has been causing you suffering. You are more

than your mind (and thoughts), and taking steps to reduce stress and radically reduce mental and emotional overload is essential for your well-being. Speak and think about your mind positively: "feed it" richly through what you reflect on, "take in," and make your own. *Use your creativity to enlist freshness.* ("*Could I look at this—or myself—somehow differently?*") Creativity is a precious gift of human existence, as your whole mind is.

Jon's story of using his creativity—or discovering it—is one that moves me and may inspire you. In his words:

I'm a mid-30s architect who thought his "creativity" was strictly three-dimensional. At Uni I had panic attacks that made exams a kind of torment. In my final year, I tentatively discovered positive visualizations. At first, they weren't much more than seeing myself somewhere relaxing. Later, I could envisage myself in any tough situations in considerable detail ahead of time, kind of deciding as I went what direction I wanted to take and, really, what outcome I was aiming for.

There are several benefits: 1) I can now "re-direct" scenarios that ignite old fears, mainly of "not making it" competitively; 2) I'm aware now of where fear takes me; 3) When I'm not calm enough to shift perspective internally, I go walking. Not sitting, not brooding, may be the last thing I want to do, yet having pushed myself out the door I can guarantee breaking the circuit at least somewhat. Funnily enough, it's my feet pounding the ground that helps most, my feet moving, getting me somewhere.

2 | Your name is not Anxious

*Anxiety is not fixed by anxiety . . . I used to get
anxious ABOUT anxiety. In order to get over it in my
experience you have to reach a point where you break
that loop. Where you don't fear or stigmatize yourself.*

MATT HAIG

Whether anxiety is with you always or erupts only from time to time, it helps to know that of all the familiar psychological challenges, *anxiety is the most treatable.* This is because you can effectively learn to put anxiety in its place, *in large part by seeing yourself more generously and your inner resources with greater trust.*

Everything this book offers supports that.

Anxiety *is not now and never will be the most important thing about you.* Your name isn't Anxious. Anxiety is *not* your identity. What's more, anxiety is never your whole "story." Nor should anxiety dictate the stories of who and what you are. Ever.

To write this book, I had to catch up on some of the exhilarating progress neuroscience has made and is still making. This is new frontier territory that affects us all. Yes, your mind is far more than "brain." Yes, you are far more than "mind." Nonetheless, brain and mind are powerful influences on your self-understanding.

To help myself as well as you, I needed to understand far better how you physiologically and psychologically respond to experiences in the present; how you store and make memories; and why some situations keep tripping you up. I also needed to understand how changes in the way you view, see, limit, or encourage yourself can best restore hope—and choice.

Science offers discoveries to support everyone enduring long-term visits from anxiety. These insights certainly include the effects on every aspect of your health when you are subjected to extended periods of stress and elevated levels of stress hormones, like cortisol.

> *Managing stress is not optional.* **Managing the physical effects of stress is also not optional. Stress does not explain the whole of the complex anxiety story. However, the release of stress hormones affects your entire body-mind. Sleeplessness, irritability, and increased anxiety can follow elevated stress hormone levels.**

"Managing stress" in a world that causes so much stress takes skill and courage. But it must be done. In *The Myth of Normal*, Gabor and Daniel Maté write that on the "terrain" of economic achievement (for some, not all), ". . . we find many people in a state of chronic uncertainty and loss of control, subject to stress-inducing fears that translate into disturbances of the hormonal apparatus, of the immune system, and of the entire organism."

That statement means a couple of things. None of us can shop our way to peace-of-mind success, believing that the next acquisition (or round of applause), or the next one, will "do it" for us. Plus, you need to know—and many, many of us don't know—that whatever anxiety you feel, it is never "all in the mind." *It is everywhere in your body.*

It makes you reactive, probably irritable or angry, and certainly tense. That affects your outlook, at least as much as your "outlook" affects your moods. Nothing in this story about you and anxiety is linear; it's all "circular," which made me feel excited when I could confirm the obvious: that when your mind is agitated, and you most identify with the emotions that anxiety brings, *soothe your body first.*

That again means strictly limiting and controlling stress—even and especially when you are saying, "That's impossible . . ."

It is also powerfully reassuring to learn more about your brain's capacity to "heal itself." This broadly means that patterns of response in the brain are more "plastic" than previously assumed. This is terrific news for anyone with a brain injury or a disease like Parkinson's. But new hope is echoed for many more people when you understand what *lets you change patterns in your thinking and responding.*

Insight depends on allowing yourself to challenge some familiar assumptions, and revise what you have been consciously and unconsciously telling yourself about yourself (and about every experience coming your way). The power of story is not just something that writers and readers know: the *"default position" of the brain is "storytelling."*

It is completely natural that you and I are always telling ourselves stories. (You also have stories coming from your unconscious in your dreams.) By "stories," I don't mean fiction or fantasies, although they may be a lovely part of your imaginative life. "Stories" are the reflection of your own evolving expectations, as well as what you have been trained and conditioned to expect—or be repelled by. They go to the heart of what you believe matters most, how you identify yourself and what you are most strongly identified with. How you inspire yourself, what you are inspired by, how you set your intention-compass for the day: all these gifts owe much to "story," even the fundamental message, "Yes, I can do this."

A need for story is deep in your human nature. (Scientists are not exempt. Science tells many stories—most of them evolving.) A need for *rich* stories is also real, stories that acknowledge your complexity, inner contradictions, slow or swift changes in perception. No one, for example, consciously thinks, "My name is Anxious. *My primary identity is anxiety. Or fear.*" But someone may well have a hundred reasons why they cannot take a risk, cannot trust anyone—even an old friend. Maybe they feel too afraid to contradict their boss at work or their partner at home. Or are regularly awake at 3 a.m. scanning their mind for things that are "sure to go wrong."

Nothing has more power than the stories you are telling yourself about yourself, about the impact others are having on your life, about what is fair or unfair, what is manageable, or not. Only some of this is conscious.

You inevitably have unconscious inner drives that can be tricky to "own." You may also be projecting—*which means you are attributing motivations or intentions to other people that come from your mind, not theirs.* Such stories—inner narratives, dramas—can be utterly convincing. They can cause severe disruptions in your most intimate or dependent relationships. Yet they are one possible interpretation only, perhaps driven by old patterns of self-criticism or worse, rather than the reality-check audit ("Is there another, kinder way of thinking about this?") available to you when you are less stressed or distressed.

Many of us who are psychologically affected by anxiety are physiologically affected by trauma, grief, fear, and anxiety.

During those hard times, your inner stories will almost invariably become blaming, floundering—and anxious. But—and it's a consoling "but"—you are not stuck with any limiting patterns, stories, or expectations.

I love it that in his core book, *The Brain's Way of Healing,* psychiatrist and psychoanalyst Norman Doidge points out that as new as some of these neuroscientific discoveries are, the insights about your essential cooperation with your whole-self healing are ancient.

Dr. Doidge writes, "The father of scientific medicine, Hippocrates, saw the body as the major healer, and the physician and patient working together *with* nature, to help the body activate its own healing capacities."

No matter how intrusive anxiety is in your current life, it need not and must not define you. Nor need it dictate the stories that consciously and unconsciously guide your life. Truly, however you identify, whatever you most identify with, *your name is not Anxious.*

3 | Step back from anxiety

*To be yourself in a world that is constantly trying to make
you something else is the greatest accomplishment.*

RALPH WALDO EMERSON

One of the most useful skills I learned in my early years of therapy training was how possible it is to *disidentify* from beliefs and attitudes that may seem fundamental to your identity and sense of self yet seriously dent your self-trust and engagement with life.

The very idea of loosening those largely unconscious identifications was radical then, and now. It basically means discovering more consciously what's going on in your own mind about how you see yourself. And also discovering that you have the capacity *to step away*, emotionally and metaphorically, from patterns of thinking or assumptions that are trapping you.

Loosening the hold your very own thoughts have on you is already a jolt. Then there are those scenarios you are running and rerunning, plus musings, reflections, inner dramas. Oh, and those inner criticisms or instructions that seem so natural. Or inevitable. Or "authoritative."

How can it be possible to stand back and recognize, "I have thoughts. I am more than my thoughts"?

There's nothing unusual about being closely identified with your own thoughts. And states of mind. But when a particular state of mind dominates, it is worth investigating. As with all the best insights, you will need to explore this for yourself, finding as you go that *the same mind that seems to trap or trip you sometimes is also your greatest power and resource.* How so?

> **You and I have a marvelous capacity to observe what's happening in our own world of thought,** *except when we are in crisis or overwhelmed by emotion.* **At those times, quite different methods of self-care are needed, and needed fast.**

In better times, and always in a spirit of curiosity and experiment, pausing and observing, or just reflecting on the patterns of your thinking, you create crucial distance between yourself and the states of mind that are in any way limiting you. *You take back the power that's rightfully yours. You are less compelled; you have more choice.*

I was barely thirty, living a pressured life in London—my home for most of the previous decade—when I first heard the term "disidentification." At the time, I knew—but didn't want to let myself know—that I was hugely overidentified with making a success of myself as a young publisher.

My sense of self and self-worth went up and down with my work success. I worked obsessively hard in a career I loved (after early years of study and work I did not love). But I also gave away to others much of my power to define myself. I could not take difficulties in my stride.

I was a perfectionist and often harshly self-critical. I would rehearse how I would cope when/if things went wrong. I gave myself too little chance to enjoy what was going well. (Familiar?)

Most of the people in my social circles were also seriously concerned, as I was and am, with the health of our world. We were active on our own and others' behalf. But even when we were waking up to those vital connections between our outer and inner worlds, I would say that discussions about depression dominated, and anxiety was far less recognized. This was true even when anxiety was driving self-sabotaging behaviors like eating disorders, severe social anxiety, or the anxious perfectionism that I was experiencing. We saw anxiety more like being nervous, worried, jittery, concerned about *something*, rather than as a state of mind and being that affects the way you perceive, trust and value yourself. We saw how anxiety around self-worth persuaded many women, especially, to put themselves down harshly and unfairly. And how racism and sexism affected millions daily, holding them back from their full potential.

In the years since, anxiety has become far better understood—and needs to be. It has reached plague proportions in our world. The statistics are alarming. You, though, are far more than a statistic.

It may be little or no comfort to view anxiety as an entirely rational response in a world where the climate is changing at unprecedented rates, where we now know that pandemics change as well as cost lives, where work is unstable for millions, where the gaps grow ever wider between the hyper-rich and the devastatingly poor, and the "future" seems to have arrived at a bewildering pace. *Yet tragic is not all that our world is. And anxious is not all that you are.*

Knowing what I now know, I would have identified my own

psychological struggles more accurately and much earlier. I had suffered not just grief but trauma in my childhood when my mother died when I was eight and she was in her thirties. No one talked about children's grief. No one understood the lifelong consequences registered in the brain and body as well as in the unconscious mind. I was creating a sense of self-worth through my work because I had little or no sense of an anchor within myself. And I certainly don't believe I was confident in finding an "anchor" in or through another person.

"Overly" concerned with the world's woes, obsessive, high strung: none of those descriptions is generally offered as a compliment. Yet to my mind, when not running feral, they—and a manageable degree of anxiety—also keep me closely in touch with *life*, with other people's suffering and the compassion they need, with the grieving, the wounded, the lonely, the disappointed—as well as with the beautiful, blissful, and beauteous. In short, with the rich complexity of our human family in all its width and depth and mystery.

> **That phrase, "when not running feral," is a telling one.
> Bit by bit, and sometimes in a rush, anxiety invades our
> consciousness. It shapes the stories we tell ourselves,
> especially the stories about who we are and what we
> can or should expect from other people. This can
> deceive us into thinking anxiety and enduring chronic
> stress is normal, however debilitating it may be.**

Anxiety can become so entrenched in your psyche that it becomes the prism through which you view yourself and experience the world. You might hear yourself saying, "I can't do that, I'm too anxious . . .

I'm having panic attacks just thinking about . . . I can't sleep at night for fear that . . . I hate the very thought of . . ."

Such statements don't only describe someone's anxiety. They describe a lack of confidence in that person's own inner strengths and resources. And an identification that is deep with what's wrong, what's been wrong, and what might likely yet go wrong.

In almost every workshop I have run in whatever country, I have heard some participants putting themselves down, expressing some of the thoughts that fuel a lack of inner security and may even keep them in a state of heightened stress that has serious effects throughout the body.

This is not because those people lack emotional intelligence. On the contrary, they are often among the most committed, caring individuals you could hope to meet. What's likely is that they are expressing habits of thinking and feeling that they have had for so long they have come to believe these thoughts—the innermost stories they are telling themselves—are self-evident and "true."

The processes of identification, even with something as unwelcome as anxiety, may have been lifelong. They are often born from trauma and lodged in the amygdala. The strength of their power is likely unconscious even when anxiety is all too consciously felt.

A far more vigorous and generous self-awareness lets you recognize how you have been describing yourself to yourself—and how you can take charge of that. (That's the work of self-therapy. Or should I say, that's the adventure of humane, self-loving self-therapy.)

We are all creatures of habit. You. Me. Every one of us. Until we get a needed jolt, we won't even consider doing something differently. Yet how freeing to discover you can! Years ago, after an injury, I had to switch from using my right hand to move the mouse on my computer to using my left. Could I do it? Not easily, but having no choice was a powerful catalyst.

Habits are only habits. Have fun with this. Experiment. Sleep on the "other" side of the bed. Swap responsibilities with a partner or colleague. Don't "always" switch on your television first thing after dinner. Check what you say you could never do. Perhaps you could? Your spirits as well as your brain love to be startled. "Dance the orange," says poet Rainer Maria Rilke in one of his sonnets. Defy convention!

By learning to detach at least somewhat from any stories or reactions that might be diminishing you, you can assess their effect. You can discover that *these are habits of thinking and feeling*—that need not determine your future. More self-encouraging, self-caring habits can and will shift the way you see yourself. For the better.

That change alone is massive.

4 | Putting anxiety in its place

I was born and grew up in a colonized country, Aotearoa / New Zealand. I now live in another colonized nation, Australia. For a decade and a half in between, I made myself thoroughly at home with former "colonizers" (sorry, Britain!).

Chronic anxiety is also a "colonizer," taking possession as if by right. The more powerful it becomes, the less powerful you feel. It can trick you into believing constant crisis is the new normal, and that living with stress, distress, and anxiety is inevitable.

If that's happening to you, you need to "decolonize" yourself: switch the power balance. *Claim choice.* That's the core of what I offer here. And I'm confident that it is possible. In fact, I believe it is more possible than it has ever been, despite anxiety reaching plague proportions globally and robbing millions of us of pleasures and adventures, as well as easy good humor and relative calm.

My trust that you can put anxiety in its place—at least most of the time—comes from a recognition that, for the first time in human history, you can draw on the wonders of neuroscience as well as workable psychology.

Your "mind" is more than your brain functions. "You" are (much) more than your mind. Nonetheless, understanding something of the intricate biology of anxiety can steady you and make sense of what's happening inside you that's feeling difficult or impossible to regulate (a word that psychologists love). Before I do that, though, I want to say, loudly, that *having strong feelings doesn't mean you are weak.* It means you are passionate. Expressing those strong feelings—as well as experiencing them—is healthy.

Who would not wish to care, love, grieve, mourn, rage, or yearn with heart and soul? However, when "strong feelings" are driven by fear, *conscious self-care* is needed to lessen the pain and panic.

Fear and chronic anxiety are whole-body experiences. They are not *just* emotional reactions. Your body-mind has evolved to protect you from danger, but it cannot effectively protect you from your own constant thoughts of danger—and the physiological effects such thoughts arouse. These include the release of stress hormones that can cause irritability, weight gain, gut problems, headaches, sleeplessness, poor memory, high blood pressure—none of which soothe the body or help anxiety.

Strong stress reactions are also related to trauma or painful experiences as a child where you had little or no control and virtually no means "to save yourself."

Stress hormones have more effect on your whole body than the better-known fight/flight/freeze reaction. Chronic stress affects you in so many different ways, with lasting neurological and physiological consequences that inevitably affect your spirits.

**If you are emotionally stretched or feeling fragile,
you may be flooded with "I can't cope" feelings.**

Or you may be saying, "This is all too much."

**And it is—far too much, unless you have
some clue what's going on.**

Getting some sense of your "emotional brain" is highly relevant to those of us with strong imaginations. It is here you generate your never-ending stories, running the equivalent of mind-movies. ("Those of us with strong imaginations" is everyone who can conjure up the painful, worried "thinking" that sustains anxiety and lets it run feral. In other words, me—and maybe you?!)

The "thinking brain" gets a lot of credit for the more considered judgments you make, for looking at the big picture, for giving others the benefit of the doubt, for owning your part in things. *And for giving you a chance to respond in supportive ways to complex situations, rather than "flying off the handle," or "losing it."*

The prefrontal cortex is where you develop vital executive functions like working memory, planning, prioritizing, initiating, as well as responding flexibly. That doesn't happen fully until you are in your mid-twenties. Meanwhile, teens and younger adults are processing information far more emotionally. (Who can forget this? Or the recklessness that can mark those teen years and into our twenties? I am not exempt.)

It's tempting to make some jokes about those whose "thinking brain" never seems to switch on, but the reality is that anxiety undermines all those functions. Also, *there are deficits in ideal functioning in all of us, whatever our age.* That's because what even neuroscience cannot describe or measure *consciousness as well as conscience*: a chosen response, rather than acting out, plus your stunning capacity to observe your own thoughts and *choose a different direction if that is needed.*

The interdependencies of brain, mind, consciousness, and body functions are complex, nonlinear, and near miraculous, in my view. The idea that some people keep their anxiety in check by being purely "rational" is a fantasy. It's much healthier to be aware of inner conflicts and contradictions, and to face them.

> **Observing your thoughts and the emotional scenarios they provoke is your best chance to get clarity and choice. There's no mystery to this.**
>
> **Shut your eyes, pause, and let yourself *notice* your thinking—and especially familiar patterns. Thoughts come . . . but *they also go.***

This is not something you want to be doing when you could be living fully and unselfconsciously. In fact, *live as unselfconsciously as you can. Be absorbed by life. Encouraged and even exhilarated by what life can bring.*

TRY THIS
The same mind that has caused you problems is also your greatest resource. It is a shift in "seeing" that is needed.

1. Check on the assumptions you are most often making—especially when they are driven by difficult events that have already happened—or may never happen.

2. Let yourself know what's needed—if anything—*in this present moment*, including soothing and reassuring yourself.

3. Do more of whatever brings you into a positive connection with yourself, others, life.

4. Make a commitment to "check in" regularly by compassionately observing your thinking—and where it is taking you.

5 | What is a "whole self"?

A whole self is you. It's me. It's everyone on our wondrous, threatened, awesome planet. It's *who we are*, always something more than whatever label is put upon us, or that we accept or create for ourselves.

A whole self is mind, body, spirit, instincts, memory, imagination, consciousness, shadow, light, past, future, present—and so much more than I could list. A whole self is a concept. Even more, it is an experience that's complex—and simple. Coming to see myself as a "whole self" has been lifesaving for me. It has allowed me at least two transformative insights:

1. That every single one of my experiences adds up to who I am and who I am becoming; that I do not need to split any part of myself off from the rest—including my worst mistakes or deepest regrets; that *my healthiest and most healing drives are toward wholeness.*

2. That I—an evolving "whole self"—am also *part of a greater whole that we call Life*. I will never fully understand that greater whole, which—for me—extends beyond the material, measurable universe. This sense of unconditional belonging—to our world, our human family, to the

greater whole—grounds me when I might otherwise drift. It lets me know I am *part of things*. I recognize that my choices and actions affect others. I know their choices and actions affect me, and that our responsibilities (and delights) are collective as well as individual.

Protecting ourselves from other people's judgments is a painful aspect of contemporary life, made worse by rampant competitiveness. And perhaps by social media giving us too many chances to offer airbrushed versions not of who we are, but of how we want to be seen. What we don't want "seen," or to see, can be unconsciously disowned, shoved into what Carl Jung names as the "shadow." From his *A Little Book on the Human Shadow*, poet Robert Bly explains the shadow neatly: "[The shadow is a] long bag we drag behind us . . . We spend our life until we're twenty deciding what parts of ourselves to put in the bag, and we spend the rest of our lives trying to get them out again."

How you are seen (and judged) is a major source of uncertainty and anxiety for almost everyone, whether this is acknowledged or not. It goes beyond status and body anxiety. It goes to the crux of *who you are* in someone else's eyes—most of all if you are unsure of *who you are* in your own eyes. Unpicking this with love is essential. Perhaps also with tiny, powerful phrases of self-acceptance when otherwise self-critical habits might creep in. *You are a unique human being, whole, and with a part to play in the wholeness of life that no one else can fulfill. No one but you can be you.*

It helps to genuinely understand what blocks that healing depth of self-acceptance. For some it is a lack of self-worth. For some it is the cruel judgments of an ignorant society. For some it is the tormenting messages or voices in their own mind. In my inner world, perfectionism trailed me for much of my adult life.

This extra degree of self-acceptance helps me to be less anxious about "things going wrong" or making "terrible mistakes." *Things will go wrong, of course they will,* whatever my best intentions. More helpfully still, holding on to this concept of a whole, evolving self has given me back a healthier sense of proportion. Big events deserve a big response. Some things—many things—can pass on by.

Treating yourself like a friend, with understanding and without too much tension, makes it possible to acknowledge and draw on your inner strengths and values, your invaluable lived experiences, your precious wholeness.

I first heard this term "whole self" at a simple yoga class held in the bare living room of a house in a bushy suburb of Sydney. This was fairly soon after I arrived to live in Australia, and years after beginning my therapy odyssey. As directly as the words "whole self" pierced me, I had to take the concept in slowly. I had to comprehend in my deepest being the extent to which I had cut aspects of myself off from conscious understanding. I needed to understand that when I blamed myself for my own inner insecurity or suffering, I made it worse, not better—and that a kinder way was possible.

With time, I also had to acknowledge that even the professional success that I was "giving my life to" was not necessarily going to offer me the inner stability or reliable self-worth I yearned for. When I began to notice my life as a whole, rather than piecemeal, I could see how it was sometimes my most glittering moments of "success" that left me feeling hollow and unreal—and more rather than less anxious about future achievement.

Who am I apart from my achievements was a question that I couldn't answer only by doing better. This form of perfectionism or performance anxiety frequently goes with an absence of sensed "wholeness," and an absence of self-trust. This affected my relationships as well as the way I connected to myself—or failed to. The imbalance between doing well and feeling empty was particularly stark. With time, I had to find self-forgiveness for the countless times I pushed myself in unhealthy ways. And for when I had projected my anxieties about doing things so-called perfectly onto other people, making their lives harder than they needed to be.

I needed to discover—slowly, slowly—how to look at myself through the eyes of understanding, as well as forgiveness. And accept that this shift was more than psychological. It comes down to what you believe is the meaning of existence, why you are here, what most matters. What brings spirit to your living. What brings peace, as well as excitement. Are we spiritual beings on a human journey? It has helped me to believe so. Others are sustained by learning to discover and trust that what they need, they can find: through the kindness of others, and through the bigger challenge of kindness to oneself.

Little by little, I had to learn to see the people I love and the people I don't love as whole selves, too. I had to use this concept to shape what it means to me to be a mother to my two now adult children, by far the most important role I have had to learn as a single mother (from their middle childhood) whose own mother could not be with her, or them. I had to use this new notion of trusting a bigger sense of self to take on subject areas in my writing life where I felt unworthy or unready, despite intense years of research and experience.

Perhaps more surprisingly, I had to learn that a lightness of heart can, and, perhaps even must, coexist with seriousness of mind. I had to tame my self-criticisms and fears of what life can and will bring. I needed to learn the gentle arts of self-encouragement that could change my attitude *toward myself*—and, I believe, make me easier to be around, as well as making it easier to be "me."

6 | Discover the power of self-therapy

A moment's insight is sometimes worth a life's experience.
OLIVER WENDELL HOLMES

Insight and action are the yin and yang of self-therapy, and that's what this book is offering. Taking ourselves seriously and doing something about what's holding us down or back is essentially empowering. And therapeutic. This is a book of self-therapy drawn from decades of experience showing me that out of more positive ways of viewing your life you can discover more self-trusting, more enlivening ways of caring for yourself (and all your relationships).

High levels of anxiety make clear thinking next to impossible, not least because they cause you to regress, losing touch with your hard-earned adult maturity and making it hard to keep your moods steady—or even to make familiar, easy decisions.

Many people bluster or lash out when they feel pushed. Some become paranoid and desperate to find fault with someone, anyone. Some collapse in a heap. Some have gut problems, back problems, asthma, skin rashes, or addictive behaviors around food, alcohol, gambling, overwork, sexual or physical risk-taking. None of this is easy. *All of this can be addressed.*

Self-therapy is a way of seeing what's helping or harming you. And doing something about it. It gives you a self-respectful, insight-filled, and creative means of reclaiming power over your own life rather than having anxiety run your life for you.

That means going beyond self-soothing or making yourself feel a little better *right now* (as helpful as that can be). It means feeling stronger *from the inside out*, and less dependent on other people's reassurances. It means changing the foundations of how you see yourself—most of all when those "foundations" have become shaky.

In her book *Unf*ck Your Brain*, Faith G. Harper defines anxiety as "a state of full body disequilibrium at a level of intensity that demands immediate attention and corrective action on your part. It can be in the face of a real or perceived threat, either present or anticipated." That's a definition that I can certainly relate to. "Disequilibrium" may show up in feeling agitated within yourself, as often as you feel vulnerable and stripped of resilience. Or highly agitated about and with the personal world around you, and uncomfortably reactive to it. (Also, hard to bear.)

When this goes on and on, it steals your confidence as well as your peace of mind. You need more than a Band-Aid. Rather than looking at your recent or past experiences as evidence of "everything going wrong" or "feeling awful" or "feeling out of control," self-therapy lets you *use your own experiences to gain insight*, especially around situations that may frequently be tripping you up.

Insight and power are not all you get. Self-therapy turns those ah-ha moments into attitudes, actions, and behaviors that can *enhance every aspect of your well-being. You can break habits that harm you. You can shift to a more generous view of others, as well as yourself.* You can achieve those significant changes in your own way and time.

> **Self-therapy gives you the means to care differently and better. It actively honors the countless experiences *you have already had*, rather than discounting them. It lets you realize *how much you already know*, and what strengths you already have.**

Positive insights about yourself—that self-therapy gives—diminish anxiety's power. They shift you away from feeling defensive or reacting fiercely to a situation that feels frightening, unjust, or out of your control. Positive insights give you a bigger "view." They rebuild resilience, experience by experience. Beyond their effect on your mood and emotions, they influence the way you hold your body, how you literally face outward to the world, what you are willing to express without or beyond language.

Self-therapy might more accurately be called "whole-self-discovery." It shifts the emphasis from what's "wrong," to a broader, deeper understanding of the person you are. Self-therapy—on every page in this book—needs and *develops* your imagination, your creativity, as well as your insights. "How could I do this differently?" is such a basic question, yet so easily neglected. Guided self-therapy—being offered here—lets you find that out, in *your* way, for *your* life, meeting *your* needs.

Self-therapy does not take the place of professional support when that's available. What it does do is allow you to use the breadth of your own experiences—and a better understanding of them—to live with a more generous attitude toward yourself, your life, and how you are consciously and unconsciously directing it.

Self-therapy doesn't need to replace support you may be getting from your social circles. That can be complex to accept when you feel vulnerable. Or angry. Or overwhelmed. Self-therapy helps with that. How? Because as you become more self-aware, and less controlled by your moods or fears, you will very naturally feel more open with and appreciative of other people. You can let them in at least a little bit, accept their clumsiness and imperfections—as you learn to accept your own. Connection and contact are human needs. Anxiety can leave you stranded, alone, feeling like no one understands you. As self-therapy brings you into a better relationship with yourself, that will ease the way you view others, not as potential "judges" or as sources of irritation, but as everyday people as much in need of encouragement as you are.

Self-therapy enlarges your thinking and, therefore, the way you describe situations to yourself and react to them. It supports every aspect of your well-being and every aspect of your life. *And it is always available.* However well you are supported—or not—you are in your own company 24/7. That's where self-therapy can give unique encouragement, and the confidence that emerges from it.

Whatever form anxiety takes in your life, and however much power it seems to have over you, using self-therapy to help yourself has an immediate double benefit. First, you will experience that there's much you—and only you—can do to bring greater equanimity and resilience directly into your life. Second, in experiencing that you can make changes for the better, you will regain the vitality that anxiety has eroded.

My experience of self-therapy—and my trust in it—goes back to when I was a young professional, living in London and discovering how urgently I needed to deal with long-suppressed childhood grief and an entirely premature, partial independence that circumstances had forced upon me. Despite appearing confident and charging ahead in my beloved publishing industry, I slept badly, worried fiercely, and was overly dependent on "doing well" to justify my very existence.

This was a time when therapy was having a dramatic renaissance, with a quite new emphasis on the inescapable effects that social and cultural influences have on each of us. My first experience of personal therapy was in London with a caring, sympathetic analytic psychotherapist who most sincerely wanted to help me—but could not. In fact, we spent so many hours sitting in fairly desperate silence while she waited for me to speak that I mostly felt worse after our twice-weekly sessions, and rarely better.

Her way of working was dependent on unearthing the buried or unconscious emotions that might hold someone back in their relationships and how they feel about themselves. This required me to re-experience devastating feelings of loss and trauma that I had repressed since childhood, while not taking me forward to integrate those feelings with a sense of wholeness as well as self-compassion.

Her training meant that my therapist paid little or no attention to the parts of my life that were going well. Or very well. *My strengths and coping mechanisms were not part of our conversation.* Nor were tools or actions to change behaviors. It took me more years of different therapy experiences, plus therapy training and, later, many years of self-accepting spiritual practice, to really "get" that as profound and life-shaping as my most wrenching experiences were, they are a part of me—and not my whole self. I had feared drowning in those sorrows if I let them in to my more conscious mind or spoke of them aloud. Such fear was itself threatening, and that traditional psychoanalytic way of working aroused the helplessness of a motherless child without bringing into the picture the flourishing in my adult life, beyond survival.

Around the same time that I was first in therapy, I commissioned in my work as a publisher what became a magnificent book called *In Our Own Hands*, by Dr. Lucy Goodison and the late (and much-missed) Sheila Ernst. Not only were those writers determined to share some accessible skills and insights that can help us, but they also wanted to challenge the idea that only a professional can give us back an inner steadiness when that's diminished or even lost.

Sheila was a hugely talented therapist herself, and both women ran groups and workshops that benefited hundreds of people. But they knew—as we still know—that grief, trauma, and anxiety affect your body and spirit as much as they do your mind. They also knew that adequate therapy is not always available, that many people can't afford it, and that some of the skills can be learned and creatively used by "us," for us, and for our own individual and collective benefit. *They demonstrated, too, how empowering it is to gain insight and translate it for yourself into action. Human life is dynamic. Self-therapy can reflect that.*

Years later, after I had trained in both analytic psychotherapy and in a psychospiritual psychology called psychosynthesis, and after I had begun to make writing my primary work, I continued to keep self-therapy as a central value. I saw it then and see it now as a workable, creative, and sometimes inspiring way to connect to yourself. And, out of feeling better "understood" and freer, to connect with greater ease and acceptance with other people.

TRY THIS

Regard any strategy here as an experiment. YOU are the expert in your own life. See how and what works for you. Shifting from familiar ways of limiting yourself is tough; it is also strengthening. Insight is your friend. So is a positive intention.

Setting a strong, self-respecting intention leads to *positive action*. "My aim here is . . ." Or, "I have nothing to lose by . . ." Or, "I'm ready to experiment with . . ." Or, "I'm taking charge of . . ." *Commit a positive intention to paper in no more than a single sentence.* Perhaps put it in an obvious place where you will be regularly reminded that power for change is in your hands if *you choose that*. (This also "wakes up" the *initiating functions* of your thinking brain, which is itself empowering.)

Anxiety is wickedly persuasive. It catches the most caring and thoughtful of us. That makes it worth a daily reminder, "Anxiety is not who I am. Anxious is not my name. I am a whole self—in discovery mode."

7 | More than your thoughts

Thoughts can be utterly persuasive, especially when they are "yours" and strong emotion comes with them. But how many of your thoughts are fresh? Or interesting? How often do you challenge your familiar assumptions, especially when thoughts roll over into judgments of yourself or other people? Or when thoughts become tyrannical, loading you up with admonishments about what you should be doing or what kind of person some inner or outer authority requires you to be?

So much of what passes for education is about rote learning and not inquiring. *Thinking about thinking benefits us.* So, I was delighted to discover how much our brains apparently welcome being startled. (Not frightened, but given a shake-up by considering something new—excellent "brain therapy" at any age.)

Great poetry can startle you, and so can a vigorous exchange of ideas, a work of art, or deeply looking at or into something awesome in nature. A sensual moment of delight is a wonderful way to be startled. So is rethinking a familiar assumption that is weighing you down. So is discovering that something is so ridiculous or hilarious you are laughing out loud.

Taking in enough new information to "startle" your familiar assumptions demands a willing openness of mind. This is fine when you are excited about life and are thriving. It becomes harder if you feel ruled by anxiety and are more in survival mode.

To explore your own patterns of thinking, it helps to consider thinking as something you do: *it is not who you are.* You may well "live in your head." (That's been me for much of my life.) You may value your intellect above anything else. (Hmmm, maybe me there also?) Your greatest pleasures may come from "thinking activities" like reading, talking, or writing. You may even be aware that your brain never stops "thinking" and "telling stories" even when you are sleeping (and your unconscious is prompting you via dreams). And what are stories but a series of thoughts and ideas, impressions and assumptions, strung together?

For all that, though, "you"—a whole-self "you"—are more than thinking, however constant or profound. You are more than feeling, instincts, memories, body systems, brain, mind. And without getting into metaphysics and worrying if "more" adds up to spirit, soul, life force, or mystery, you can simply experience that *"you" can observe your thoughts—even while you are having them.* Clinical psychotherapist Tao de Haas wryly and correctly says, "When you notice you are experiencing anxiety, *the part of you that notices isn't anxious.*"

This is the insight that gives birth to multiple insights. It is the basis of all mindful meditation practices that are at least 2,500 years old. I would venture to say it's an insight as old as consciousness, because that's what you are exercising, an "awake" awareness that you have thoughts that *are not all that you are.*

How is this relevant for those of us who are at a hyper-expert level when it comes to worried or anxious thinking, who can swiftly and in great detail imagine a dozen scenarios, each one grimmer than the last? *It is wholly relevant.*

Experiencing that your thoughts—and especially your patterns of thinking—are not inevitable, not all-powerful, not with you "forever," and not defining you, is radically freeing from ways of thinking that may be limiting or even bullying you.

This is not a mysterious process. *You have an innate capacity to observe your own thinking.* Nor does it require you to be a skilled meditator, or any kind of meditator. Or to stop thought (you can't). It simply asks that you pause, go inward, and observe.

Pause and observe (your own thoughts) to loosen the idea that your thoughts are something that can push you around, frighten you, put you down, or make your sense of self far more fragile than it needs to be.

It also lets you ask the ridiculously helpful question: "Is there another way I could be thinking about this?," opening your mind, yourself, to go beyond stuck feelings toward the possibility of something fresh.

If I have not made this clear enough, I so wish we could sit together at this very moment, for I have never met anyone who suffers chronic anxiety or depression who does not suffer from their own thoughts—and there's a kind of tragedy in that.

Your magnificent mind should be a source of creativity, curiosity, strength, and wonder—and it can be.

Anxious thinking—A-grade worrying, which is my speciality, driving a kind of obsessive perfectionism where I can only fail—will not disappear. The volume, though, can be turned down. Other possibilities can arise.

Your inevitable storytelling (self-talk) can gain a new tone. A bolder "view" and understanding is needed, plus the courage at least to experiment with the idea that thoughts are inevitable—*yet are not the key to your identity.*

> "I have thoughts. I am more than my thoughts."
> "I have feelings. I am more than my feelings."
> "I have instincts, memories, opinions. I have
> consciousness and imagination. I am more than
> all those precious aspects of being human."
> "I have regrets, sorrows, griefs. They are part of who I am.
> They are not all of who I am."

Memoirist and popular novelist Elizabeth Gilbert has written, "Your emotions are the slaves to your thoughts, and you are the slave to your emotions." *But you need not be!* Without becoming in the least bit robotic or overly detached, you can loosen the hold that habitual ruminating patterns have on you. You can observe, experiment, and notice that no matter how convincing those thoughts or ruminations are, or how intense the feelings they arouse, *no feeling or thought is permanent.* They are dynamic, just as you are. Dynamic. Changing. Evolving. Alive. Just as you are.

8 | Conducting your own chorus

One of the loveliest writing commissions I have ever had was creating the libretto for a short opera. Writing is generally an unhealthily solitary occupation (which may explain the broodiness and moodiness—and ubiquitous anxiety—of many of us writers). So, when I do have the rare chance to work collaboratively, I grab it.

Given what a delight that work was, I felt like quite an impostor when people's responses to "I'm working on an opera . . ." seemed overly generous. I knew the real credit went to my close friend, musician/composer Kim Cunio. It was he who wrote every note for every instrument and every singer. He had to make a whole of the many parts.

Our opera, *Rising*, was commissioned in response to dramatic floods in the Australian city of Brisbane. In the years since, climate change has brought even worse flooding to many parts of our world, including Australia, the "driest" of all continents.

While music has always been a love of mine, my love for it outstrips any talent I may have. What I learned from cocreating *Rising* was how essential it is that a skilled conductor knows each instrument and voice, knows when each should come forward or recede, knows when "singularity" is called for and when a grand "uniting" should prevail.

In your mind and mine, there are many voices. Thoughts, "stories," sometimes feel like instructions or orders. This is certainly true for people who suffer from auditory hallucinations. It is as true for those who have, for example, a strong Inner Critic, or an inner Harpy doing its best to pull you down and shut out the far kinder words of self-encouragement you might long to hear.

To call them "voices" may only make sense to some of you, but just imagine for a moment what you are likely to "hear" within yourself about a situation when you are feeling "on top of the world." And how different that commentary will be when you are feeling "in the pits."

In *How to Survive the End of the World*, British writer Aaron Gillies notes, "The anxious brain doesn't just jump to conclusions, it polevaults over them into a new territory of ridiculousness. Your worst fears are projected into your senses, and when it comes to relationships, betrayal is a common paranoid symptom. Anxiety can leave you helpless, a victim of your own over-active imagination."

You may assume that, voices or not, your inner commentary is something you just have to put up with. I want to challenge that. With a kind of internal "stepping back," you can observe your own thoughts, and even pick out a couple of familiar inner "voices" to test the quality of messages they bring.

The first may well be your Inner Critic. The second could be the Harpy telling you that you shouldn't, you couldn't, you can't do whatever it is without falling flat on your face and making an absolute fool of yourself. (I had a therapy client who called these voices "Mean" and "Scary." I liked that.)

Noticing is key here. You may be used to being convinced by negative, dispiriting messages arising within your own mind. They might feel natural. You may suspect they are half or wholly right. Some detachment is essential before they begin to lose their power. And if you find the whole idea of conducting your own inner chorus quite ridiculous, all the better. Humor and playfulness support your creativity; they don't diminish it. Perhaps it will be a while before you can ask, "Is that the Inner Critic whining away?" Or perhaps, "Should I listen to the Harpy telling me what I can't do?"

You are the conductor. Voices are only voices.

9 | Meaning and purpose are lifesavers

Life is not primarily a quest for pleasure, as Freud believed, or a quest for power, as Alfred Adler taught, but a quest for meaning.
VIKTOR EMIL FRANKL

One of the most fascinating discoveries made by outside researchers in Okinawa, where an extraordinary number of people lead vigorous lives up to and past the age of one hundred, is that most of those people practice a philosophy called *Ikigai*, which overtly values community, engagement, meaning, and purpose derived not from anything abstract, but from the attitude you bring to your everyday tasks and living.

Living is itself meaningful—especially when it's not done on autopilot. *Meaning and purpose are not optional extras in a busy life. They are life.* Appreciating that brings a depth dimension to the most unassuming existence. It makes getting up every single day worthwhile.

**Nothing is more precious than your
desire to live—and to live fully.**

If stress, anxiety, depression, or your social circumstances take that desire from you, it will need all your courage to restore it.

Suicidal ideation is on the rise, along with anxiety and depression. It is that, more than anything, that drives me to try to find words that may help to restore hope, if that has been lost. There is scarcely a philosopher or "clinician of the soul" who has not addressed the agony that looms when someone loses touch with their will to live. (I am not meaning here someone finding acceptance in the final stages of a terminal illness, but rather someone who is well enough in body but fragmented in spirit or mind.) This loss is at the extreme end of anxiety; nonetheless, it can coexist with any significant loss of connection and joy, and certainly with a loss of purpose and meaning.

Viktor Frankl is a shining hero of mine. He has been a profound teacher in my life and in the lives of millions of others. His most famous book is *Man's Search for Meaning.* That short, life-changing book came from Frankl's experiences in four death camps of the Third Reich, including Auschwitz. Under some of the worst conditions humankind is capable of creating, Dr. Frankl—as a neurologist and psychiatrist—was able to observe how vital *meaning* is to sustain a desire to live, even when your conditions of living seem increasingly impossible to bear.

Today, "impossible conditions of living" may be far less grim than the death camps, yet may still be outside your control. It may be the cruelty of poverty, homelessness, displacement, loss of work or health. Or the profound miseries caused by violence and war, or the injustices we see everywhere on our planet.

A possible loss of meaning—and the will to live—may also be caused by other people's behavior, as with humiliating bullying or prolonged abuse in a workplace or, worse, within your own family. *If your home is not a place of safety, external help is basic to your self-care.* A loss of meaning can certainly follow psychological or spiritual pain or trauma, most particularly when this extends into an indefinite future. "Nothing seems to matter anymore" is a cry from the soul.

Meaning cannot be understood as simply answering the question, "Why?" It was Sufi poet Mawlana Jalal al-Din Rumi who wrote: "The eye goes blind when it only wants to see why." On anything but the simplest issues, simplistic cause-and-effect thinking seldom takes us far.

In the face of serious or acute suffering, meaning must be discovered, rediscovered, not imposed.

Frankl believed it invariably connected us to something bigger than ourselves—not "God" necessarily, but a sense of connection and purpose that brings each person more securely into life.

> **Even when your life is not in crisis, having some understanding of what gives your life meaning is indispensable to well-being. That's because *it is meaning that connects your past with your future.* It is integral to your sense of being "you," whatever else is going on around you.**

Many in our human family fill their lives with a hectic round of activity in order *not* to face the question, "What gives my life meaning?" It is almost ironic that some of the most familiar distractions from finding meaning and purpose decrease well-being—even when that's the last thing you want. When your life is paused by illness, grief, or any significant setback, including anxiety, that pause can become an opportunity to think freshly about meaning—and *your freedom to do so.*

Viktor Frankl founded a therapeutic approach he called logotherapy. This literally means "therapy through meaning." It was his belief
that humankind's drive for meaning is greater than our drive for power
(as Alfred Adler believed) or for pleasure (as Sigmund Freud taught).

Frankl's theories run counter to the kind of nihilism, superficiality,
and meaninglessness that produces so much greed, or indifference to
others' suffering. Or tragic hopelessness in the face of your own suffering. A drive for meaning may be strong in your life—even if you have
never considered it in this way.

**For many sensitive people, or those suffering the anguish
of persistent anxiety, a discovery of "therapy through
meaning" can be life-changing or even lifesaving.**

I give a powerful contemporary example below, but one of the
most moving examples of the transformative power of greater meaning comes from the years of Dr. Frankl's own therapy practice in the
United States, where he went as a refugee after the Second World
War. In his role as psychiatrist, Frankl was visited by an old man, a
medical doctor, who told Frankl that his wife had died two years before and that he (the patient) was stuck in a grief so profound he could
not overcome it. We can imagine how carefully Frankl would have
listened because one of his key principles is *not* to compare "your"
suffering to another's but to respect the dignity and humanity of each
person who suffers. (Not saying, "You think you've got problems! Just
wait until you hear about mine!")

So, what was Frankl's response to his patient? He consciously held
back from offering any kind of interpretation but instead asked the old

man a question: "What would have happened, Doctor, if you had died first and your wife had to survive you?" The old man responded with a passionate sense of how terrible that would have been for his wife. At which point Dr. Frankl said, "You see, Doctor, such a suffering has been spared her, and it was you who have spared her this suffering—to be sure, at the price that now you have to survive and mourn her."

This account from Dr. Frankl tells us that the old man, the widower doctor, said nothing but shook Dr. Frankl's hand and left his office calmly—in contrast to the agitation he had expressed earlier. Frankl writes, "In some way, suffering ceases to be suffering at the moment it finds a meaning, such as the meaning of a sacrifice."

I can share another example of the simple, profound power of identifying meaning from my own time as a psychotherapist, although in this instance I was asked for help in my role as a minister. The woman in front of me (I'll call her Kristina) was thirty-seven, the same age my own mother was when she died from cancer.

Kristina's suffering was obvious to me from her extreme loss of vitality. She had a major depressive illness with visual hallucinations that frightened her even when they were benign—like seeing cats where there were none. She also suffered from a persistent loud voice she called the Inner Tyrant, rather than an Inner Critic. This Inner Tyrant was feeding her hideous lies about her life's intrinsic value and worth. It was a loud, persistent voice she could not silence.

Kristina couldn't sleep. She couldn't rest. She couldn't feel any pleasure. She was switching between feeling fiercely angry and desperate or collapsing into hopelessness and despair. Do I need to say that her anxiety was off the scale?

Kristina had a caring therapist and was on medication prescribed by a competent psychiatrist. She also had a loving, involved, caring family. But she wanted to see me as a minister, even while she had, in her own words, "Little or no reason to believe in a miracle that would end this." Her temptation was to discard the "miracle" she could not hope for and "end this" by ending her own life.

You may not have experienced despair or hopelessness on this scale or witnessed it. Or perhaps you have? Either way, I want you to imagine the courage it took for her to tell me, someone she knew only from my books and a single workshop, and the immense courage it took for her decision to remain open despite the incalculable weight and persistence of her suffering.

I owe everything to my faith in Dr. Frankl's logotherapy that I was able (just) to bear my own fears for her by asking her less about her illness and more about her three young boys, and the circumstances in which she is raising them. The details are hers and not for me to share here. However, it was clear that one of those sons, Jacob, is a soul as sensitive as Kristina is. Taking my cue from Frankl, I asked her if she was confident that this child would recover from the death of his mother.

This was an agonizing question for me to ask and no doubt more agonizing still for Kristina to contemplate. I can say with absolute truth that I have lived a long, rich, humane life. But did I "recover" from the death of an intensely loving, accepting mother who was my rock and safe place? Have I experienced any sense of "getting over it"? No, I have not. Even now, do I carry with me a heightened sense of responsibility that is extreme and unachievable and hugely anxiety-provoking—because I, a child, could not "save" my mother? Yes, I do.

My question to Kristina had to be direct. "Will Jacob survive your death, especially if he knows it was chosen?"

Then, in the face of her silence and anguish, I again found the language that the "therapy of meaning" gives us. "However great your suffering is, you are bearing it with love for your three sons, and especially Jacob, *in order that they will grow into adulthood with your love to protect them*. Each day you choose life *for love of them* is a day of profound courage and accomplishment. It is also a day in which the greatest possible meaning is not just understood. It is lived."

Part Two

Emergency measures

10 | First, calm your body

Not everything that is faced can be changed, but nothing can be changed until it is faced.

JAMES BALDWIN

Your most important act of self-care is to avoid getting to a crisis point. At that time, your stress hormone levels will soar—and you will inevitably feel far more anxious, sleepless, irritable, with less access to your working memory and "thinking brain." Take it for granted that you cannot afford to ignore the stress responses in your body-mind that will inevitably make anxiety worse.

And when you have reached a crisis point?
Calm your body first.

When your mind is telling you there is danger on all sides and your very existence is threatened, *your body will react brilliantly to protect you.* This works well if you need to escape a life-threatening situation. Hormonal and physical changes let you "run for your life." These bodily reactions don't work as well if it is your own complicated feelings and perceptions that feel endangering. Or if your stress levels are on permanent high alert. The rule then is simple: *calm your body first.*

Take it for granted you won't feel like doing what's needed when it is needed most. Your anxious mind will protest. Your panicked mind will . . . panic. You may hear yourself telling yourself and anyone else that any remedy is stupid, a waste of time, won't work, is hopeless. That's why preparedness is so important. Preparedness means facing it, just as writer James Baldwin expresses in the quote at the start of the chapter.

If your mind and psyche are vulnerable, then understanding what is happening in your body—and learning that you can stay in "charge" by calming your body—is self-therapy at its finest. *Taking positive action on your own behalf is a necessity.* Decide in advance what your emergency measures will be. Practice them daily when your *anxiety is not at crisis point.* And every day, *every day,* look for ways to reduce stress.

If you feel suicidal,
YOU MUST CALL AN EMERGENCY SERVICE
or go to your nearest outpatient facility or emergency room.
Whether you want this, or whether it's the last thing you
want, regard this as a medical crisis. That's exactly what it is.

When the crisis is less acute, there is a great deal you can do to help yourself—and to help anyone supporting you.

Understand *what's happening in your body* when your anxiety is acute. That is essential. It is certainly not something that I in any way comprehended for many years, despite headaches, upset stomachs, skin rashes, no appetite or too much appetite, and decades of poor sleep.

When you are very anxious or stressed, you won't be capable of clear thinking or good decision-making. You may feel regressed, childlike, detached from your grown-up self. (In many ways, you are.) *Your levels of stress hormones are going up.*

You may not feel that you are breathing fast, but it is highly likely you will be breathing quickly and shallowly.

> **The more elevated your stress hormone levels are (and for longer times), the more "stressed" you will feel, not to mention sleepless, agitated, and irritable.**
>
> **To calm the body in a real way, *you must address what causes you stress—as well as the effects of that stress.***

If the emergency is *now*, you may want to try the more dramatic intervention I describe in chapter 11.

Where the situation is less urgent—and however resistant you may feel—discovering how to pay attention to your breath can become your own effective emotional first aid that is available to you at any time and wherever you are.

Slow, focused breathing can help. It tells your body, "The crisis is over or passing." All the danger-meeting instincts and systems can slow down. Yes, you are using your mind to help your mind. You are also using your mind to support your body, discovering as you go that mind and body are integral.

Decide on a breathing practice well ahead of when it is needed to help you in a crisis. Direct your breath to a more centered place within the body as you slow it. Counting ONE in/out breath up to TEN in/out breaths is steadying. It not only slows your breath. It gives you something to focus on. When you get to TEN rounds of in/out breaths, then start again. Gradually direct your breath down into your trunk, into the base of your spine, into your legs, feet, the soles of your feet, breathe into the place where your feet meet the earth, even when there are socks, carpet, floor, between you and the earth. (How long should you continue? My strong suggestion is that you do this twice a day for five to eight minutes when it is for your general health and benefit. When it is a crisis, I would suggest you do it for three to four minutes, take a very short break, then repeat for three to four minutes until you feel calmer, more inwardly "collected," more like yourself.)

You may prefer to give your body a cold shock. I write about that in following chapters. Some people I have worked with go running, working with their body's speed—but that is not for everyone.

It may be hugely tempting to go further into what is psychologically tormenting you. *This is not the time.* You may not be having a panic attack, but treat yourself (and your severe or accelerating) anxiety in much the same way. You need to signal to and through your body that you are managing this so that your cortisol and other stress hormones—made by your adrenal glands—do not further flood you and make the situation worse.

**Stress hormones have a more powerful effect on the
body than the fight/flight/freeze impulse. When
anxiety puts you under constant stress, the high levels
of cortisol in your body cannot return to normal.
This intensifies anxiety.
This robs you of sleep.**

If you have a medical doctor supporting you, you will know if emergency medication is called for. Make sure that the people around you know what is happening physiologically. Being told to "just calm down" is not helpful. Nor is being ignored or shamed.

Action to protect yourself needs to be swift and effective. This is also most definitely NOT the time to cause or engage in a fight.

It is NOT the time to further disinhibit yourself with alcohol.

It is NOT the time to make decisions of any consequence, however tempting or even "logical" they may appear.

Most seriously of all, this is NOT the time to decide whether your life has value. *It does. It does. It does.*

You may also need to talk soon after a difficult time or even while it is happening. There are mental-health phone services that meet this need. *It is self-caring to use them.*

Understanding that you can help yourself—that you can be supported, that you are not alone, that your body is doing what it should (though not as often and not for as long), and that this will not go on forever—is experiential wisdom, lived wisdom, at its very best.

You *can* be kind. You *can* be your own best supporter. You *can* get through this.

11 | Adjust the temperature when needed

This is the very best emergency method I have so far discovered—and one I learned not from anxiety causing my body stress, but from *my body causing my mind stress.*

For some very uncomfortable years, I had problems with the "electrical systems" in my heart. The heart itself was, according to the cardiologist I regularly saw, "pristine." Whatever regulates heart pace, however, was way out of kilter. Frequently, and toward the end of that period, almost every day, my heart would begin to race and in moments be up to 170, 180, 190, or even 200 beats per minute (bpm). Your heart, and now mine, should be at about 60–100 bpm.

This feels horrible. It is frightening and exhausting. The condition itself is called SVT (supraventricular tachycardia). What's even more sobering about the condition is that the "cure" for a cardiac ablation, where deliberate scarring is caused in order to halt unruly electrical impulses in the heart, was not generally available until the 1990s and may still not be widely available for all who need it.

The first ablation that I had didn't work. The second one did, but in the long year between the two attempts I had to learn to leap out of bed or up from wherever I was and undertake what are called vagal maneuvers. These sometimes troubled me almost as much as my racing heart. However, they did give me some power to slow my heart rate. This mattered because, on the few occasions when I couldn't do this, I had to go to the hospital where my heart was fleetingly stopped then started again. (No picnic.)

Some vagal maneuvers involve breathing out strenuously while bearing down. What worked most effectively for me was dunking my head into a basin filled with ice and icy water.

This was something my pediatrician husband had used with heart-racing children (it's less commonly used by adults). Vagal maneuvers trigger the vagus nerve to act positively on your heart's own natural "pacemaker." Interestingly, the vagus nerve runs from your belly to your brain and is a major influence on your parasympathetic nervous system.

Why am I sharing this with you? Because it was not for a few years after my successful second ablation that *I discovered how vital the parasympathetic nervous system is in relaxing your body after intense periods of stress.*

Acute anxiety and panic attacks, overwhelming obsessive fears, the inner conflict that prolonged tension causes: all of these are bodily states made worse by stress and likely to intensify and prolong it. (Don't confuse this with the sympathetic nervous system, which controls your body's fight/flight/freeze responses and which, for some of us, may be on call 24/7.)

It is immensely helpful when it comes to self-care to know that the parasympathetic nervous system does something called "downregulating." It uses the vagus nerve to send impulses from the brain to the body *and* back from the body to the brain.

To my surprise, *I discovered that my parasympathetic nervous system informs my brain about what's happening, rather than my brain directing my body.*

This supports heart function—as it did for me. It may also support less stressed, calmer emotional well-being and overall physical health. Some researchers have suggested it could possibly influence a longer lifespan. Both mild exercise and conscious relaxation, including meditation, support your parasympathetic nervous system. *All are worth exploring for overall, everyday well-being.* This is practical self-therapy. It is also excellent self-care.

TRY THIS

If you're agitated, defy "hopeless" and try one of the following:

Start with a brief warm shower, then run the water as cold as you can bear to make it. Focus on the feel of the cold water on your body—even if it is less than a minute initially. Enjoy the shock! Open your mouth to gasp and to take in some water. Don't think; *feel*. Feel sensually, feel part of the water. Luxuriate in being one with the water. You may want to end by warming yourself up, but it's the cold water that is most benefitting you. Rub yourself down with a towel, noticing the physical sensations that take you into your body and out of your head.

Alternatively, use the vagal maneuver that I did, dunking your whole face into a bowl of freezing water and stay there until you feel like your lungs might burst. Surface, gulp some air, and go under again. It won't be comfortable! It may feel shocking. But it is profoundly distracting and will send a message to your nervous system(s) to slow down.

This second technique is also used in DBT (dialectical behavior therapy) to de-intensify stress or overwhelming emotions. It is called "the mammalian dive reflex" and can be used if you have a panic attack or feel as if you can't control your anger or sadness. (I am not talking about grief here; that's something quite different.)

This is something that you can choose to do to take control of your own anxiety or stress. *It is not something to impose on another person, ever, for any reason.*

A final thought: until you have tried a technique like these—and found it helpful—*it is unlikely that you will want to do it when you need it most*. Mid-panic, mid-rage, mid-despair, these ideas will make little or no sense to you. Hopelessness will take over.

When my heart was racing crazily, I had no choice but to do everything I could to bring its beats per minute close to normal. Your situation may, however, be different. And may *seem* less urgent. Your self-care action may be just as life-changing.

Decide *when you are calm* that you are willing to try this—especially when you do not feel that controlled or whole-self breathing will be enough.

If you have a companionable, supportive partner, family member, or friend, discuss it with that person. Explain that this is about *getting your body to help your mind*. Then, when a crisis moment hits, you can effectively help yourself.

That knowledge, as well as the experience, brings trust back to where it belongs.

12 | Swim cold, feel well

The idea of throwing your body into freezing water—either into a swimming pool or the ocean (if you are lucky)—can seem more than daunting. (Are you shuddering at the thought of it?) Yet increasing evidence shows that immersing your whole body in cold water and exercising—not simply standing in the shower—is the kind of positive, side-effect-free "shock" that can be of real and lasting benefit to your mood and outlook.

There is probably more research and discussion about cold-water swimming as an antidote for depression than for anxiety. For many of us, the two are intertwined. Certainly I found clinical studies suggesting that "anxious depression" is linked to higher rates of suicidal ideation than some other forms of depression (like melancholia). "Anxious depression" also expresses itself in irritability, psychomotor agitation (repetitive or involuntary movements), and a restlessness that may well be exhausting while preventing good sleep.

No treatment is a guaranteed panacea for everyone. It may be tempting to try this once or twice and then say, "It hasn't worked for me." I am wondering, meanwhile—and this is a choice entirely for you to make, ideally in consultation with your therapist or doctor—if it is worth a reasonable trial if you know your psychological story includes anxious depression? Or if you and others know that irritability (or an anger flare) is a warning sign when your inner world feels most oppressive?

For centuries, people in the Nordic nations have combined sweating in saunas and rolling in the snow! But I am *not* recommending swimming in icy water; far from it. If the cold shock is extreme, there are risks, including neurogenic cold shock or hypothermia.

"Cold" is a subjective experience; perhaps water that takes some effort to get into is cold enough for "winter swimming."

One study suggested "that winter swimming abolishes general tiredness, boosts self-esteem, and improves mood and/or general wellbeing." That's quite a claim.

On this and so much else, the "Middle Path" is advised by Buddhists, walking the road as the historical Buddha did between extreme asceticism and extreme indulgence.

This applies in so many situations, including cold-water swimming. How exhilarating, though, if you were to discover that even a short dip—a few minutes only at first—can work for you. And that the greatest expenses are a wet suit if needed, goggles, and either the entry fee to your nearest pool or a bus ride to the ocean.

13 | An ocean-swimming story

The following first-person account comes from Nicola Sage Gardener, an artist and writer living in a rural town in Victoria, Australia. Cold-water ocean swimming has been transformative for her, and after five years she is fully committed to its benefits. I asked her to share her story. *I follow her story with some necessary words of caution.*

These are Nicola's words.

Most days I experience some, if not all, of the following ailments: mild headaches, emotional instability, grumpiness, anxiety, muscle tension, and general aches and pains. Most people would be advised to have assistance from some form of medication. However, since I took up ocean swimming five years ago at the age of sixty-three, I still experience these ailments but to a lesser degree, and after a swim my symptoms are gone and not to be felt again until the next day. Now I spend most days ailment-free. I swim every day and this routine has become part of what I do for my well-being.

In the ocean I go through a daily transformation, a dimension of bliss and a spiritual experience as well. The ocean has become my friend and a true friend indeed! She gives me relief and healing. When I am totally immersed in Mother Nature's liquid, I experience the pleasure of her healing hug.

I swam alone for three years, and two years ago decided to share my experience of ocean swimming with others. I started a swimming group called "The Numbskulls," an apt name I think for Victorian waters where water temperatures can go as low as forty-six degrees Fahrenheit. My favorite water temperature is around an invigorating fifty-seven degrees Fahrenheit.

To swim in the ocean every day does take a certain amount of determination and courage, and there will be some obstacles to overcome.

1. Fear: The ocean is very powerful and to feel afraid is to have a healthy respect for the ocean and her cycles. Like any friend, it takes time and effort to become familiar with her changing nature.

2. Cold: I see the cold as just a different bodily sensation from heat, only one is invigorating and the other dulling. I now feel the warmth in the cold and love the tingling sensations. As I don't wear a wet suit, and depending on water temperature, my general rule is twenty minutes in summer, and ten minutes in winter. Moving around in the water is also important. (Make sure you rug up well immediately after swimming, especially in winter.)

3. Rain: Unless there is a storm, there is no reason to stay home. You're already going to get wet swimming, so a little rain is not going to make you any wetter. I love swimming in the rain.

4. Salt on your skin: Many people seem to fear that salt on their skin will make it dry. I rarely shower after a swim, and if I do, it's because my hair may need washing. I have discovered that my skin does not dry from salt but from the chemicals in tap water. Also, by not showering you allow

the ocean's healing minerals to be absorbed through your skin. I choose minerals over chemicals.

Nicola's enthusiasm is contagious. For her, there have been significant benefits in well-being. Those without access to an ocean might choose to experience a few moments under a cold shower each day for the adrenaline spike it can bring.

> It is important to emphasize *this is not medical advice.*
> It is also not a test of how "tough" you are. If ocean
> swimming is to be part of your regular routine, and
> not used as I used ice water (on my face only) to reset
> the parasympathetic and sympathetic nervous systems,
> *it is essential to check this plan with a medical doctor.*

A final word: Do *not* undertake cold-water swimming on your own. A "shock to the system" can be gloriously invigorating; it can also be dangerous.

14 | Irritability. Overwhelm. Anger.

Have you overreacted lately to something trivial? Have you felt put-upon by someone just asking how you are? Has someone else's clumsiness or slowness driven you mad? Are you flying off the handle where once you wouldn't have? Is anger the most passionate emotion you feel?

It's vital for your self-respect as well as your well-being to know that anxiety affects all of us neurologically. It affects your perception and mood. It "disorders" and deregulates your complex nervous systems—and your reactivity can go sky-high. This adds to your distress. And the out-of-control feelings that are all too real can be as destructive of your relationships as they are of your own well-being.

It's probably inevitable, after all, that when you are chronically tense, overalert, sleep-deprived—and anxious—even quite ordinary interactions between you and other people will begin to go badly.

You may feel easily hurt. You may be quick to snap at others. Or feel crowded by their mere presence. You may discover that your resilience pot is empty or that you are angrier than you have ever been.

Outbursts that are angry or critical of others will *make your life tougher.* None of us wants to feel that our emotions are running the show. We all hate "losing it" and the painful effect this has on others.

No matter how anxious you are, you will want to manage the pressures and stress that are so much part of contemporary life. Yet, as your mood plummets, your vulnerabilities increase. *This is because major pressures from the "inside" make any additional stress from the "outside" so much harder to bear.*

I understand this. I live with chronic pain. I have had periods of serious though not life-threatening depression. Anxiety around caring adequately for others has been a low or louder hum through much of my life. What I have also discovered, however, through my own experiences and through talking to many people about their anxieties, fears, and dreads, is that when you feel most vulnerable to painful and potentially harmful emotions, you are almost certainly pushing against stress rather than finding ways to relieve and diminish it.

It is vital to understand that when you are anxious, depressed, or in chronic pain, you will quickly be drained of energy and vitality. This is itself a state of stress. With those losses, your usual resilience will disappear.

You may react strongly to minor setbacks. Disappointments may feel like wounds to your fragile sense of self. Pressures and further stresses become unbearable. The smallest extra demand is "too much."

This is not an excuse for behaviors that are "unlike you." But once these issues are acknowledged, they can also be addressed.

Tension and stress are both major energy sappers. So is anxiety. When your mood is low and/or your anxieties are high, the energy you lose is both physical—made worse by brutal disruptions to your sleep—and emotional. It's exhausting to feel at odds with yourself and your social world. It increases your vulnerability when that's already shaky.

If you do find you're routinely snapping at others or seeing all their faults in Technicolor and none of their good points, if you are infuriated or overwhelmed by ordinary daily demands, that's because you are emotionally drained as well as agitated. This will affect your thinking.

The cognitive effects of stress and anxiety are real and probably well-known to you. You will quickly become sensitive to real or imagined blows. You will find it hard to look past something that's stupid or careless but not meant to hurt. Where there is unkindness, your vulnerability makes it difficult to see that as a reflection of the other person's pretty troubled inner world, not of you. Injuries will hurt. They will also quickly add up.

You may find it harder than ever to make decisions. And you might torment yourself about whether they were the "right" ones. Your focus and concentration suffer. How could this not make your experience of anxiety worse? So does your memory. A long period spent in any inner state of disharmony is a major stress, made worse when ordinary daily demands pile on top.

As grim as all that is, these distressing reactions clearly tell a story—especially if such behaviors are "not like you" in better times. Any or all of them can let you know that thoughtful, self-caring action is needed. Not "sometime." Or when you "have time." *Now.* (Or even sooner.)

Bonnie is certainly not a lone voice when she tells me, "I can honestly say that I have felt the loss of self-control around my emotions and moods as more painful even than the loss of health that comes with long COVID."

Bonnie's story struck me as particularly poignant because she had been a senior theater nurse before catching COVID. In her late thirties when she was infected, she expected to get through the period of isolation and resume a normal life. Like millions of others, that wasn't to be.

The neurological effects of long COVID are measurable and alarming. So are the "energy crashes" people experience after even quite mild exercise. These are due to nerve dysfunction, often in the autonomic nervous system, which affects breath, digestion, and other crucial body systems. Some of this will sound familiar to those with chronic anxiety, bringing gut disturbances, perhaps dizziness or a racing heart and breathlessness. Bonnie continues her story.

I had periods of depression and certainly some panic attacks in my teen years. I know I was awful sometimes to my parents, but as I am the youngest of four, they put my rages and rudeness down to teenage hormones. Correctly, I feel. While I was studying and certainly for the years I worked in surgical units, I'd say I was pretty calm, considering it's a stressful environment. I was also really social. That's gone now.

These last couple of years I have lost my confidence, my profession, my sense of self. I can't help that. Maybe I can't even help having such bad anxiety, and I am getting treatment for that. Where I feel like I have really "lost it," though, is in the emotional arena. Angry? Bad-tempered and critical? Yes, yes, and yes. Feeling like I am both exhausted and jittery, so I could fly apart at any moment? Certainly.

The effect on my friends and family has been the hardest. My partner has somehow stood by me, but nothing about our relationship is the same as before. It is not long COVID. It is long COVID creating a worn-down version of my old self—with the new "me" lashing out, no matter how often I resolve to do better.

If you feel easily irritated, hurt, or insulted, you may recognize yourself in some part of Bonnie's story. But her story does not end there. Nor does yours. *Anxiety, loss of energy, "brain fog," and a major disruption to your moods and powers of thinking go hand in hand. So do the remedies.* Experience will show you that reacting to other people critically, angrily, or with frustration compounds your existing problems. Other people will avoid you. Or tiptoe around you, driving you even more to distraction.

At the moment you feel most powerless, you have a choice. It takes insight, then bags of courage to acknowledge that your *reactivity or moodiness affects other people.* Yet making changes for the better, you will bolster your sense of self *and* improve all your relationships. For many of us, that is a fine place to start. *Own your behaviors.* That means noticing when your reactions are causing you or others hurt—and apologizing for them. It also means discussing with people closest to you that this is something you are working on: reducing your anxiety, plus the pressures affecting your moods. (When your cortisol levels are high, you will find it difficult to sleep and you will likely be irritable. It is essential—not optional—to reduce stress.)

TRY THIS
- Check all the causes of stress in your life—and ruthlessly monitor them. Where the stresses are economic or have to do with something as fundamental as having a safe home or somewhere to live, *seek and find help. Feeling the anxiety plus the stress is always too much.*

- Identify any obvious reactive patterns that *may feel entirely justified* yet are making your situation harder. ("I find it worst when someone's crowding my space. It feels as if they want to criticize me.")

- Check if there is often an "all too much" moment, and what was going on just before it.

- Notice when you feel particularly vulnerable. *Or most triggered.* This may happen around the people you love most, yet also have the most complex feelings about. Talk honestly when you can about what they—and you—can do to help.

- Avoid people who have hurt you badly in the past. If they are still in your life, minimize your contact and do not allow any discussions to become personal. Otherwise, limit your communications to texts. (Or get help to manage this.) *Being bullied is a major stressor.*

Can you relate your unwelcome reactions to your more general state of physical and mental health? To your energy levels? To how tired or exhausted you are? Can you see how much easier it is to cope when you are feeling robust than when you are not?

> *An anxious society impacts you ceaselessly.*
> **So do the stresses of everyday living. As you become
> more aware of your vulnerabilities, your anxiety can
> quieten. As your anxiety becomes less intrusive, you
> will monitor those stresses more and more effectively.**

Many people have self-help strategies that *may make the situation worse.* They can include overwork, self-medicating with alcohol or recreational drugs, or risk-taking that makes your life unsafe. They can also include excessive fitness training or even self-care like yoga or meditation when that fails to address more fundamental issues.

TRY THIS

Undertake a regular "stress audit." That means putting your emotional well-being above everything else—*and includes your capacity to consider other people.* A life empty of rewarding contact and ordinary pleasures, or meaning, needs your attention every bit as much as an overcrowded one does. *What are you making time for? What are you neglecting? Who is choosing?*

A successful check of this kind deserves your time and may additionally demand professional support. The powerlessness that anxiety brings with it may be worsened by your (legitimate) feelings that *too much is constantly being asked of you*—and that your employer, your family obligations, or your efforts to make a living are all factors that have more power in your life than you do. People who are lifelong carers of others may well feel that there is no moment to call their own. (And I am not forgetting parents of little or bigger children, either.)

Carving out some sense of agency and choice is critical here.

This is where conscious choosing of attitude is itself an action worth pursuing. I don't mean that you should be pretending all is well when it is not. Nor should you be a martyr. But finding greater meaning in those obligations can truly help (as Viktor Frankl's logotherapy emphasizes).

Try, too, reaching out and asking for help. It's brave. It's powerful. With many people living under extreme pressure, I suggest cultivating the fine art of micro-breaks. These may involve a quick nap (and why not?). But try, too, focusing on something that is natural, delightful, or pleasing to your senses, for at least five minutes. Make a ceremony of it: perhaps going outdoors to "kiss the ground" with your bare feet; perhaps looking at a familiar painting or reading a favorite poem to discover what you are seeing for the first time; perhaps a self-rewarding "tea and biscuit" ceremony—not your usual coffee, not your usual cup, but something beautiful and precious, reminding you of *the infinite value of your very own life.*

15 | Don't tell me what to do

*I went gray with frustration at the remoteness of my own
mind, my very selfhood . . . I was coming up against
a physical reality that conflicted with my assumptions
that I would, by now, be on an upward trajectory.*

MEGHAN O'ROURKE

If you are experiencing the loss of control over your life that almost
invariably comes with serious anxiety as well as depression, it's highly
unlikely you will cheerfully welcome other people's opinions, views,
or advice about what you should be doing. How you should be "dealing with this." Or what they would certainly be doing if they were
you. "This" will not be your anxiety only. It could include the grand
sweep of your everyday behavior, impulses, and attitudes.

This is tricky territory. You feel undefended. You may also be irritable, tired of your own state of mind, sleeping badly and eating not
much better, and doubly anxious because it seems like nothing you or
anyone else can do could possibly make things better.

On the other hand, you half know that your anxiety is contagious.
The people closest to you are concerned about you, desperate to help,

81

feeling inadequate to help, and awkward with it. Under those circumstances, they will almost certainly say and do the wrong thing, and you may find it extremely difficult or impossible to extend to them any semblance of tolerance, never mind the lifesaving "benefit of the doubt" that might be available when you and they are more robust.

Irritability and loss of patience follow anxiety like a shadow. You may even recognize that you are not just anxious but seriously stressed by how difficult it is to be remotely gracious, tolerant, or amenable. Especially with the people you love most.

TRY THIS
Explain how anything that remotely resembles an "instruction"—"You ought to . . . ," "You should . . . ," "Have you considered . . ." is intolerable to you. It doesn't feel supportive. It feels intrusive.

Your loved one's suggestions are likely motivated by care. Acknowledging that will help everyone—including you. In place of an instruction or anything that resembles it, would it feel better (give more power back to you) to simply be asked, "How can I help?"

When your automatic responses are overwhelmingly negative, that takes you both into a hard place. You may feel powerless. But in reality *you have more power than the person trying to say or do the "right thing." Perhaps you can help them?*

You could help them by suggesting they ask, "Would you like a hug?" Or, "Do you want space?" Or, "Would you like a walk?" rather than that person giving you a hug, retreating, or telling you how much good a walk will do.

Each of us is different. And we are not "the same" from one day to the next. What matters most is that you feel acknowledged and not intruded upon. Too many choices, "help" that's too eager or intrusive, help that comes with lots of words, will intensify stress rather than relieve it.

But the caring person has their pain also.

Acknowledging their efforts, inquiring how they are—and listening—may feel too much when your moods are lowest. Nonetheless, connection and communication remain crucial. When words can't be shared, a walk can be. So can ordering in a meal, writing the briefest of notes, offering a touch on the arm or shoulder. Even at your bleakest times, *especially at those times*, the smallest reaching out helps. Not just that other person; you, too.

16 | Anxiety is a robber . . . and a liar

Anxiety is a robber when it takes hold of your feelings. It robs you of your natural optimism and much of your vitality. Along with stress, it exhausts you. *It is also a liar,* telling you what is seldom if ever "true" about the richly complex person each of us is.

Anxiety welcomes in every harsh word or criticism but keeps out or trivializes the appreciation and encouragement that others may be more than willing to give. Unconsciously you may believe the criticism *because it fits with your fears.*

It breaks my heart to hear someone say, "I am hopeless." Or, "I know for sure I'll make a mess of it." Or, "It's not worth trying." Or, saddest of all, "I hate myself. I hate my life."

Overwhelming anxiety *is* a fierce burden to bear. Bouts of anxiety, panic attacks, sleeplessness, obsessive thoughts: none of these are remotely welcome. What's more, those debilitating states of mind have a profound effect on the body. They drain energy faster than you can generate it.

Anxiety often isolates you, making it hard to feel connected. Or valued. "I hate people," one woman said to me. Perhaps it would be more accurate if she could say, "I hate that it's so hard for me to be with people."

Fear of failure, fear of being shamed or humiliated, fear of what other people may be thinking, fear of the unkind critic in your own mind, fear of being "found out" to be "not enough:" these all express deep anxiety. So is a depth of pessimism and insecurity about your inner world—*your very self*—that makes it necessary to constantly seek or need approval or praise from other people.

We know that some degree of anxiety is a normal part of being human. We would be less caring without it. *The issue here is proportion.* And how strongly you identify with a painful, battering state of mind that seems to have taken up lodgings permanently.

"Stepping back" internally is one of the most powerful psychological tools you can use. *Even acknowledging that anxiety is only part of your vast repertoire of experience can reduce its power in your life.*

Disidentifying from anxiety and its power lets you know, again, "You have anxiety. Anxiety is just part of who you are. Your name is not Anxious."

It is equally possible to disentangle what challenges deserve attention and must be dealt with, and those that are vivid in your mind *but may never happen.* A sense of foreboding is painful to live with.

That, too, needs putting in its place. I love this quote from the famous American writer, Mark Twain: "I am an old man and have known a great many troubles, but most of them never happened."

The thoughts you have when you are most anxious "belong" to anxiety. They seldom reflect a generous whole-self perspective. You are right to question them, challenge them, ignore them.

Anxiety can rob you of less pleasure when enjoyment of life becomes one of your daily intentions. Appreciation supports that intentionality. So does engagement.

American poet Mary Oliver speaks for so many poets and for so many of us when she implores us to notice the preciousness of our lives, and that we can know suffering all too well yet still experience awe, wonder, and amazement, not in the "great" moments only but also in the subtle and familiar. Hope, I believe, is securely on our side.

TRY THIS
Reclaiming your power to choose is doubly invigorating. Especially when it involves actions, and even more when you don't "feel like it."

Reduce anxiety's clout by setting up some quality distractions. The breathing suggestions here support your parasympathetic nervous system. The cold-water shocks are basic mental health first aid.

In addition, search your memory for times when you felt calmed by a physical or creative activity—or exhilarated, or pleasantly exhausted. It's impossible to emphasize enough how moving your body and/or creative thinking *forward* will also move along debilitating moods.

What you are doing is taking charge, leading your mind (thoughts, fears, dreads) in a livelier direction than anxiety can ever take you.

Move the body—or your creative imagination—to move the mind is the simplest of mantras. It may also be the truest. Why? *Because you are choosing action over staying stuck.*

17 | Bullying is always toxic for you

Bullying is a boundaries issue. It brings cruelty into your physical space, even when it is "just" words. (Words can be vile and deeply scarring.) It also invades your psychic space, risking how you feel about yourself in the deepest parts of your being. That's also where fear lives. And trauma. *Protecting yourself is a highest priority.*

Do bullies themselves act that way because they are anxious, fearful, addicted to imagining the worst? Or do they act that way because they are projecting their own fears of insignificance or self-loathing onto others: finding fault in other people to feel "bigger" or "better" about themselves?

There are no simple answers here. Some bullies get sadistic pleasure from hurting other people. Others enjoy the self-righteous "rush" as they exert power they very foolishly believe they are entitled to have.

Genuinely humane, grown-up, thoughtful people DO NOT EVER BULLY. They do not disparage, name-call, tell harmful lies, or undermine. They do not willingly cause others to suffer. They do not take pleasure from "putting others down." They do not confuse sensitivity and compassion with weakness. They are particularly cautious around people who have less power than they do. Yes, they may sometimes be angry, even unreasonably so. They may get agitated, frustrated, irritated. *What they don't do is bully.*

Our world has far too many bullies in positions of power. They give permission, in turn, to the petty tyrants you can meet in far too many workplaces, community organizations—and in far, far too many homes.

If you are vulnerable to self-blame and anxiety, it is crucial to deflect and resist external bullying (bullying by others) for at least two very significant reasons. First, anxiety makes it likely you may be inclined to block out or question what's positive and encouraging, yet "take in" and ruminate upon what is negative and harmful. Why? Because that likely comes closer to your own worst fears. *The external bully amplifies this in ways that are intolerable. And should not be tolerated. A bully is never "right." Never.* Second, as you know, anxiety is disempowering. So is bullying. The two mixed together can defeat the hardiest among us. What to do?

> Your innate *power to observe* gives you invaluable "distance" in your mind between "you" and persistent thinking that may harm you. Experiencing this for yourself, it becomes easier to "stand back inwardly" when someone outside yourself is ranting and raving and pushing you around.
>
> "How pathetic," you might feel. Rather than, "This person has the power to affect me horribly." (A bully *is* pathetic. And endangering. Keeping yourself safe is the highest priority.)

TRY THIS

The most effective action is *inside your own mind*, refusing to give any bullying words or actions precious space or credibility. Detach. Detach. Detach. *It is essential, too, to check that you are never using hostile, disrespectful language to or about yourself.*

If you must deal with a bully in your workplace or community, do so in the company of another person who is calm, and has a clear sense of right and wrong. Be specific, with clear, recent examples. Avoid self-pity, which the bully is likely to exploit. Keep your hopes for this encounter modest. However, *you are entitled to be treated respectfully.* Make that clear. Use "I," as in, "I am finding it offensive and disrespectful when you talk over me in meetings / block my ideas / disparage me in front of others / give me vague instructions and then belittle me. How can our communications become more effective?"

If you live with the bully or share critical parts of your life, *get immediate professional help.* A bully endangers your well-being at every level. "I was only joking." "Can't you take a joke?" "You're so bloody sensitive." "You think this is unpleasant. What about when you . . . ?" *None of that is remotely respectful.* Or constructive. Gaslighting means blaming you for the treatment that harms you. *Gaslighting is an intensification of bullying.* So is any form of coercive control, including over your time, appearance, ambitions, money, and especially your way of being.

Bullies will frequently make wildly untrue assertions. "Everyone I know thinks you're . . ." In response to talk like that, I had a client who bravely said to a toxic ex-partner, "It must be horrible for you to think that way. I almost feel sorry for you." *However, you should take no risks at all when someone has little or no self-control, and you may be in danger.* Winning "points" is irrelevant. Staying safe is critical.

18 | Activate your safety net

When you are more than usually challenged by what's going on inside you, it will be essential to reach out beyond yourself, *no matter how impossible this feels*. The belief that you are completely alone, or that no one will ever understand how awful you feel, only intensifies your pain, as well as your anxiety.

Reaching out is an act of courage. It may not fix things. It may not make much difference at all, But the very act of reaching out is significant. This is just as true in periods of depression as when anxiety is running riot. *Reach out.*

Not everyone has a close person they can call on. It may need to be a professional or a mental health service. Establishing who or what will provide your safety net is basic self-care. And, as with all these self-protecting ideas, it should be done when you are feeling relatively calm, not when anxiety has pierced your defenses. When your "thinking brain" can't help you, someone else can. And must.

Ideally this will be someone who genuinely understands that while anxiety is not all of who you are, *there are times when it takes over*. Those times will pass. Those times absolutely will pass. Nonetheless, your safety is at risk here, because whenever you are seriously disconnected from your own capacities to soothe and calm yourself, you need to be able to connect to someone else who can maintain that essential trust in your well-being—while you can't.

You will not want to have to explain yourself. You will not want to have to excuse the fact that you are calling for help. You certainly don't want to risk being rejected. Whoever is your safety net person, or whatever is your safety net service, they must understand that your needs are urgent. *Severe anxiety puts all your body-mind systems on high alert even while it reduces your capacity to think clearly.*

As in any crisis, the care you need must be calming, without blame, with no demands. Basic empathy and quiet, respectful listening are what's required. And medication where that is medically prescribed.

> **Knowing you *can* call, day or night, may be enough.
> When just "knowing" is not enough, however, trust
> that asking for help when you need it is a profound
> act of self-care—and *always the right thing to do.***

In a kind of postscript, a short time after writing this chapter, I had a particularly troubling dream. Anxious dreams are a strong sign for me that there's something I need to understand better. I have two friends who are Jungian analysts, and I "happened" to be speaking to one of them about something else when I burst out with a précis of this dream. She listened. Asked very few questions. Let me see what I had missed. Then, when I thanked her profusely, *she thanked me for trusting her.* Of course, I trust her! What is even better is to experience firsthand and yet again that someone being there for us in the hardest moments helps us regain precious trust in ourselves. (Thank you, Susan.)

19 | Whole-self breathing

It was something of a surprise to me when I discussed emergency measures with therapist friends and every one of them talked about breath and breathing. Yet I know, and perhaps you do, too, that when someone is in a real crisis it can be extremely difficult for them to turn to breathing, especially when their experiences of guided breathing feels inadequate.

Slowing your breath, counting your breaths, focusing intensely on breath coming in one nostril and out the other, breathing into your diaphragm, breathing into a paper bag: These are remedies that can and do work. They will work most effectively, however, when *they are a known part of your routine*, as familiar and as necessary as cleaning your teeth, rather than something to "try" when you feel at your most fragmented.

They will also support you effortlessly when you combine simple, fail-safe breathing practices with a glimpse that you are, inevitably, a whole self (however fragmented you may sometimes feel, or if you occasionally fear that anxiety has the upper hand).

It's impossible to breathe into just a part of
yourself. Breathing consciously—"Aware that I
am breathing"—is a whole-self experience.

Try breathing only into your left side, your
right leg, your lungs but not your heart.

It can't be done.

Try breathing in such a way that it benefits your
mind but not your emotions, the open palm of your
left hand but not the closed hand on your right.

It can't be done.

Yes, you can move your *attention* very specifically.
Breath, though, is essentially integrating, and available
equally to all, whether you are famous and envied or sitting
on a park bench with all your possessions in a bag beside you.

Breathing in, *whole self*. Breathing out, *whole self*.

In a world where possessions are so highly valued, it's truly a marvelous thing to notice that no one can own the air you breathe, no one owns the oceans, the heavens, the stars. No one owns you and the way your mind works, either.

Experiment with a daily practice of *conscious noticing that you are a whole self*. And noticing that when you breathe in and breathe out—focusing only on breath—*you benefit your whole self*. A few minutes, two or three times a day, is a powerful investment in your whole-self well-being. *It is yet something else only you can give yourself.*

TRY THIS

Try any of these suggested lines. Or make your own version. Your creative variations can be endless.

Breathing in slowly, breathing out slowly, I know I am a whole self.

Mind, body, breath; soul, spirit; mortal and eternal; feelings; memories, dreams, longings; tears and laughter. And always more.

I experience breath in every part of my being.

I trust my breath.

Breath in my body, air on my skin.

As I breathe, I feel connected.

I am connected to breath. I am connected to myself.

I am connected to life.

Breathing in, slowly, breathing out, slowly, I feel peace in my body.

Breathing in calm, breathing out calm.

Breathing in . . . and out, ONE. (Repeat to ten, then start again.)

20 | Know your limits

It takes insight to recognize where your psychological or physical limits are. It takes insight and reflection to recognize those limits *before rather than after* you tip over the edge into chronic anxiety, exhaustion, or collapse.

The phrase "nervous breakdown" is used far less often than it was. Versions of it still happen, though. And to all kinds of people who have lived in circumstances that are beyond their enduring.

It could be a central part of your identity to manage, cope, get on with things. Perhaps it's a desire to be valued? Perhaps it's crucial to valuing yourself to be there for others. There is so much that's good about that, until it becomes more important than noticing that your basic self-care is slipping; that you are "too tired to sleep" or too agitated; that you are paying obsessive attention to trivia rather than sitting down with your loved ones to watch a hundredth rerun of a favorite movie, or taking time to listen without distraction to your children or a friend. Or doing what you most love—but no longer have time for.

Anxiety badly affects your judgment. It can make you tense and reactive. It can also make you frazzled so that your coping ability disappears with your good humor.

Knowing your limits and checking your priorities are essential to remaining positively connected to yourself. And that is essential to remaining positively connected to others. Does anything matter more?

A long-time London friend told me that, after a lifetime of academic success, he had to decide to abandon his scientific research and his chosen identity as a "top researcher," because the competition in his field for research grants was killing his joy and wrecking whatever confidence he had left. Another older friend recognized partway through his specialist cardiology training—for which he had "slaved," in his words, to get in—that the life and unceasing pressure were undoing him. Status? Yes. A very good income? Yes. But a way of life? Perfect for others, not for him.

Those choices are self-evidently privileged. Both men would recognize that. They would also, though, point to the huge sacrifices of time, effort, and money to get to that point where they turned away. And I would agree with them.

For anyone, at any stage of life, a feeling of constant pressure and the tension that comes with it will—sooner or later—feel *too much*. It is indeed too much. The physiological effects as well as the psychological ones are unsustainable.

You might notice an increasing irritability, or a sense of being put upon. You might be much more critical of other people as well as yourself, obsessing about the ways they are "wrong" or might now, or at some future point, fail you.

You might notice that you are living with a more intense than usual sense of foreboding. Perhaps at every moment you expect something bad to happen, or even—as with phobias and OCD (obsessive-compulsive disorder)—that unless you behave in certain restricted ways, something terrible will happen.

TRY THIS

Check which sacrifices you are demanding of yourself—and the people around you—if your identity is principally dependent on accomplishment.

We live in a success-saturated world where status anxiety rampages, and we live in a 24/7 cycle of invitation to compare ourselves (harshly and meanly) to other people.

We take on more and more. Or we give up. The famous "Middle Way" between asceticism and self-indulgence is today's "road less traveled."

Your mental health will not be the only casualty. As an overachiever myself, I know the costs, as well as the rewards. I know the heady feeling of being in the zone, rather than paying attention to what feels like the more mundane aspects of life that can wait. But can they? Can you?

Understand your own warning signs. Name them honestly. They are different for everyone. But failing to heed them is unwise—and very unloving.

21 | High stress. Low confidence.

Even in a relatively predictable life, problems of high stress and low confidence feed off one another. Feeling overwhelmed is horrible. It attacks our very sense of self. When high stress (inevitably) brings anxiety, that becomes profoundly destabilizing. Almost everything becomes harder, most especially getting organized, remembering things that are not written down, dealing with pain or disappointment, or noise, mess, chaos. Or deciding what really is major, essential, or life-changing. And what is not.

The only thing that becomes "easier" is your ability to worry. To fret. To hover over current failings and anticipate many more.

Coping is a pivotal issue here. It can be as relevant—and taxing—in the workplace as it is at home. And what an irony it is that you may hate being given anything like an "instruction" or "being told what to do," when your fears of not coping are at their worst. That means that when genuine help is offered, you may refuse it. You may even resent the other person for offering it. ("How come they believe they're on top of things and I'm not?")

It is also difficult to feel much pleasure or excitement when you are chronically or acutely stressed. Your interest in doing all the things that could make a difference can disappear fast, including everyday care like eating well, sleeping soundly, having a walk not to "exercise" but just for the joy of being outside, chatting with a loved one and giving lots of hugs. You might hear yourself snapping, cutting someone off, not listening: all signs that the stress "volume" needs turning right down. You might also turn to your favorite distractions—even when they harm you and certainly reduce your power to think clearly or act wisely.

I notice that when I am stressed (and overtired with it, or overtired and therefore stressed) I feel brittle, unprotected. That has, thankfully, gotten better with age and greater self-trust—as you would hope. Nonetheless, I can still feel "crowded" in on, flustered even about things I would take in stride at better times, and certainly inadequate to meet whatever goal or need is looming. If I didn't monitor that reactiveness carefully, I could take offense far more easily than usual.

If you are feeling more on edge than usual, it helps everyone to acknowledge that in a matter-of-fact way. *Your thinking will be affected by your emotional state.* Real or perceived criticisms from others might be mirroring the way *you are talking to yourself.* This does *not* support easy, trusting relationships. Be vigilant, too, about not projecting your inner turbulence outward. And when you do hear yourself snap, *apologize.*

When you feel pushed by "can't cope" or "not coping" feelings, you might become unfairly critical of other people, losing your confidence in people as well as in yourself.

Reducing stress (and worry) has to be your number-one priority. For your sake. For the sake of those you care about.

Regaining a more positive sense of your coping self makes a difference: to you, to others, and even to our wildly, chaotically overstressed world.

TRY THIS
Worry well. That means:

1. Evaluate any/all situations causing you stress. Is it a problem of time, of coping, of attitude, of volume? Is it what you are asking of yourself? Is it because you are exhausted? Or are you carrying past burdens you're not yet ready to put down (like resentment, or bitter disappointment, or a sense of failure)? A single "solution" does NOT fit all situations.

2. Are you worrying continuously about a chronic situation? Put some borders around that. Write out your feelings. Vent. Pray. *Take care of yourself. Never hesitate to get help when needed.*

3. *Protect your relationships. It is the best way you have of caring for yourself.* Learn how to say yes enthusiastically to whatever connects you positively to other people.

4. What would it take to put yourself and your family first in a work-obsessed world?

5. Can you honestly say what your most precious resource is? Time? Sleep? Eating well? *Relaxing?* Many people try to fit in an exercise regime, for example, when winding down may be needed. Check the "shoulds," the "ought to's," the imperatives.

6. *Practice counterintuitive thinking.* Where you feel *most competent* may

be the place to trim. Your feelings of adequacy will grow in other areas when there's less competition for your attention.

7. *Do not compare yourself to real or mythical others.* Your idea of how "perfectly" someone else is coping may indeed be true, but it could equally be that person is struggling on some front that's totally out of your view. Where you can pick up tips from someone else's apparent situation, do that creatively *to suit you, and your circumstances.*

8. Ruthlessly *determine what is essential,* and what has to wait or drop off the list. Do this with a light heart, not guilt. (Last century when people still gave frequent dinner parties, British writer Shirley Conran created a place in history for herself by saying, "Life's too short to stuff a mushroom." Find your "mushroom" equivalents. Unstuff them.)

9. Silence your Inner Critic. You are not failing. You are stressed— and taking action on that.

10. Be your own best friend. Talk about what's going well. *Praise yourself for what you are getting done.* Praise others. Praise and appreciate lavishly.

22 | Medications and therapy

If you are in crisis, it is essential to get more help
than any book, friend, or loved one can give you.

Anxiety, depression, catastrophic thinking, or suicidal
ideation tell you clearly that your highest priority is to
get back a far greater sense of security within yourself.

Nothing matters more than your health and well-being.

If you are not in crisis, but have been living for months or years with
anxiety—believing you have to put up with it—also seek and find the
best-trained, most intelligent help you can find. *It is impossible to live at
your best with chronic untreated anxiety.*

Anxiety can be treated. So can depression.

A medical doctor with experience in mental health issues is the
only person to advise you about medications. This is not the role of
your friend, neighbor, family member, a complementary health practitioner or a psychologist, counselor, or psychotherapist.

Medications are for medical people to assess and prescribe—and for you to monitor their effects, report back, and be listened to.

There is also therapy. That's where a thoughtful, respectful psychologist, an accredited social worker, or a well-trained psychotherapist or counselor can come to the fore. Any or all of those people can be invaluable members of your "team." Their support can be lifesaving. So can periods of inpatient care if you are critically unwell.

Self-care includes looking for and accepting the best care from others that you can find. And persisting against the odds if the care feels inadequate.

In the hardest times you will feel least like trying something else, or someone else. *Remember that the more unwell you are, the more regressed or foggy, helpless or even despairing you will feel.* **Take that as a catalyst.**

The value of your unique, precious life may feel entirely out of reach. That's one of the effects of depressive anxiety. *It is* **not** *an accurate assessment of you.*

Seeking adequate medical help is an act of emotional intelligence. So is using skillfully prescribed medications and working closely with a professional when that's needed. I have done all those things at a number of different points in my life.

For the majority of people, the psychological support most readily available is cognitive behavioral therapy (CBT). This can be effective, and the clinical literature certainly supports it (and the combining of therapy with medication as best treatment of all).

My own bias is toward augmenting CBT with some form of insight therapy if that is not already on offer. You need a deep picture of yourself, your griefs, your potentials. *That's the basis of the creative, interactive, experiential self-therapy offered here.* (*Talk Yourself Better* by British comedy writer and journalist Ariane Sherine is an excellent account of the different kinds of therapy and their strengths and limitations. She interviews therapists and quotes a number of people who have been patients, including, inevitably, actors and comedians.)

Therapy worked best for me when it was both support and a kind of education. I discovered that as we understand ourselves better, we are freer to understand other people, freer to respect our own and others' boundaries, and ideally freer to check our assumptions rather than jumping to grim conclusions, as anxiety often prods us to do.

That's why psychotherapists (like I was) must have intense personal therapy of their own before and while they work with others. This is not always required of psychologists.

Growing in self-knowledge—including "owning" your feelings and making your assumptions more conscious—*lifts the quality of all your relationships.* It helps you stop bringing the past constantly into the present. It stops you projecting what you assume and believe onto other people ("I know he thinks I am . . ."). Or dumping on others when you feel bad ("I hate the way you . . . You think you're so bloody marvelous, but *I know better* . . .").

Ariane Sherine speaks for millions when she writes, "I would happily kick mental illness in the balls for all the years of my life it's destroyed." In the introduction to her book, she describes her horror years, and also writes, "I would currently rate myself a 9 out of 10 for happiness. I feel that I am in the best place I have ever been, and that this is due in no small part to working on myself every week."

Andrew Solomon is a professor of psychology at Columbia University and is also a writer who has shared his mental health experiences, including in a must-not-be-missed book on depression called *The Noonday Demon: An Atlas of Depression*. Like the equally brilliant actor and writer Stephen Fry, Andrew is open about his need for medication *and* therapy. He also emphasizes our human need for connection. And for insight.

Andrew's words are just as helpful when it is *anxiety* that most troubles you. He writes, "When you are depressed, you need the love of other people, and yet depression fosters actions that destroy that love. Depressed people often stick pins into their own life rafts. The conscious mind can intervene. One is not helpless . . ."

I would take "conscious mind" to mean Andrew's observing self that can indeed "intervene." He continues, "Listen to the people who love you. Believe that they are worth living for even when you don't believe it. Seek out the memories [that] depression takes away and project them into the future. Be brave; be strong; take your pills. Exercise because it's good for you even if every step weighs a thousand pounds. Eat when food itself disgusts you. Reason with yourself when you have lost your reason . . ."

There is a strong movement—active online—that dismisses all drug therapy. Some advocates are as obsessively engaged with this as anti-vaxxers are about vaccinations. Rigid beliefs have no place, in my view, in thinking about the complex individual each of us is.

Andrew Solomon meets those views with his own: "I am often asked in social situations to describe my own experiences, and I usually end by saying that I am on medication. 'Still?' people ask. 'But you seem fine!' To which I invariably reply that I seem fine because I am fine, and that I am fine in part because of medication . . ."

23 | Talk to yourself like a friend

Sometimes it can just take a caring sentence
to jog someone in a different direction.
JAMES BROWN

Are you fearful of making mistakes, of being seen to be wrong, of not being "best," of not being "someone" in the eyes of others? Do you have vivid fantasies of falling in a heap, embarrassing or humiliating yourself? (I certainly have occasional disturbing dreams where I am anything but ready for a big occasion. Or I have misunderstood the crucial instruction. Or I have let others down. Before our family member became so ill, I dreamed that I was pounced on by a huge, terrifying black dog, even as I tried frantically to get up a steep hill, despite my poor mobility. Your unconscious can be literal. And often knows more than "you" do.)

Whenever *your anxiety about how others see you* is running riot, you may have lost touch with your intrinsic worth as a unique being. Talking to yourself harshly or cruelly can only make your inner world more painful. Just when you need to experience kindness to yourself, you are pouring salt into the wounds of your anxiety or depression. This must change.

The key to change is noticing. Then choosing. If you are telling yourself that you are a failure at everything, that your life is hateful, that your life is not worth living, then something (everything) needs a radical shake-up.

TRY THIS

Is it possible that you are speaking to or about yourself in ways you would never speak to or about another person? Are you judging yourself against standards that no ordinary person could achieve? *Do you understand how anxiety physiologically undermines your thinking/analyzing processes?* Are you prepared to speak to yourself from a far more generous, healing perspective?

1. Acknowledge the effect of *your own thinking* on your body, feelings, moods. ("I don't want to be this way, *I am harming myself.*")

2. Recognize how negative self-talk impacts your relationships. Is it making you harder to reach? Acknowledge especially how/whether you rebuff kindness or encouragement from others. ("They don't mean it . . . They're only saying it . . .")

3. Check if you are saying anything you would hate a loved one to hear or endure.

4. Check if you are particularly critical of *other* people *when your own moods plummet.*

5. Challenge anything you say to yourself that is unkind, disparaging, disrespectful—or that intensifies your pain. Be decisive. "Cut out the crap," is how nineteen-year-old Joey interpreted it. Cut out the crap indeed.

24 | Fear

The body's response to fear or stress can be stressful in itself.

JOHN A. CALL

Fear is, for most of us, worse than anxiety. Especially when it is involuntary. (There are people who seek fear for the rush it gives them. Incomprehensible to me—but my fear of fear may be equally incomprehensible to them.)

You may register fear in your amygdala—this small organ in the middle of your brain then alerts the nervous system. Nothing stays in the brain, though. Fear is experienced throughout your body, activating stress hormones like cortisol, and sending blood away from the brain to your limbs so that you can "flee" or "fight" if you need to.

Fear responses are highly developed in our species, and almost everything that happens does so outside your conscious control. It continues as long as your instincts tell you that intolerable danger is threatening you. Danger can be physical, psychological, or existential: the body registers it all as "danger" from which you need saving.

I wish that I could write about fear without firsthand knowledge

110

of it. Those of you whose anxiety tips into fear will know how all-consuming fear is, and how it is *terrifying to experience.* That is, unless it is "manufactured" fear, provoked by horror movies or terrifying rides at amusement parks—neither situation remotely comprehensible to me.

Fear was part of my childhood and continues to be one of the worst and most destabilizing experiences of anxiety that I can still sometimes have. In my childhood, my teacher mother often left my sister and me with excellent carers while she worked, and during school holidays we would spend very happy times with our grandparents.

In my memory, it was not until I was nearly seven and my mother began to spend lengthy times in the hospital for cancer treatment that I began to be not just anxious about being separated from her, but more generally fearful.

I knew my mother was doing everything she could as a young, dying woman to reassure her children. (To my knowledge, she never spoke to us about the reality that she was dying.) But I must have been terrified that she would, eventually, not come home. I do know that I was increasingly afraid of the dark and what it might be hiding. Then (and sometimes now) I would have nightmares where I would wake myself up crying out as some horror descended. Then, and still now, I cannot bear to read about or witness violence or horror as "entertainment."

Those experiences of fear are different for me in intensity—and the emotional scarring they cause—from rumbling anxiety. But they belong on the same page. When I was suffering acute pain a few years ago, I was prescribed medicinal cannabis. While it did help, especially with sleep, at the end of two years I had several hallucinations that terrified me and produced all the reactions of terror that I describe above. For me, no benefits were worth that.

Your fears may be more diffuse. Or perhaps they are all too specific? *If you live with daily fear, including of another person, it is essential to
get professional help.*

Even where your fears are largely internal, great tenderness and
compassion are needed when thinking about them. Perhaps especially
when the fear aroused is one of your own death, or of abandonment.

The sublime teacher of peace, Vietnamese monk Thich Nhat
Hanh, devotes a whole book to this topic. In *Fear*, he suggests that we
have "original fear" and "original desire" to survive from our earliest
moments of life when we enter the world as helpless and totally dependent newborns.

He writes, "Although we are no longer babies, we still fear that we
cannot survive, that no one will take care of us . . . Everyone is afraid
sometimes. We fear loneliness, being abandoned, growing old, dying,
and being sick, among many other things. Sometimes, we may feel
fear without knowing exactly why . . . As adults, we're often afraid
to remember or be in touch with that original fear and desire [to sur-
vive], because the helpless child in us is still alive."

The "helpless child" Thich Nhat Hanh evokes is felt when we
are most stressed by circumstances *beyond our control.* The phrase "I
couldn't think straight" comes into its own here.

From a whole-self perspective, compassion for those painful, involuntary responses becomes more possible when you see them as *part
of who you are*, not *all* of who you are. *You may well regress at such times,
especially when there are memory strands activated that go back to your earliest
years. But these are not marks of weakness or immaturity.*

True, compassionate understanding is needed to give yourself that essential "space" or distance between your memories, your fears, and the "coping self" you also are.

If, in the present time, you are desperate when you fear being abandoned by a friend or lover, if you are falling in a heap because your spouse of twenty years has betrayed you, if you are a "nervous wreck" at the prospect of yet more agonizing surgery, you may be tempted to feel ashamed of your own weakness, *as you are interpreting it.* You may even be berating yourself, adding additional pain to your suffering. This is profoundly unhelpful. When you experience this happening, find the courage and inner fortitude to switch the situation around.

Look at it through the eyes of kindness. Ask, "What is needed?" And, "What is stopping me from treating myself with the understanding and compassion I long to receive from someone else?"

Thay, as Thich Nhat Hanh is known to his hundreds of thousands of students, urges *careful checking to see which of our relationships are underpinned by fear, including our relationship to our own self.* Disentangling may demand support; seek it. To be connected to any situation through fear is deeply painful and can keep trauma alive.

Perhaps your fears are more diffuse? For example, what other people think about you? Perhaps you are afraid that without the key people in your life you will not survive? Perhaps you are afraid of an inner loneliness that drives you to seek out any company or highly charged experiences, rather than being with your own self?

Those fears are real. But instead of an unrealistic call to greater "independence," Thay leads us to consider what he calls the "umbilical cords" linking every one of us to all of creation. He brings attention to this very page where you are reading, or where these words are shown, when he points out that if you look deeply, mindfully, into a single sheet of paper you can see the sunshine in it that allowed trees to grow, and eventually to be harvested and transformed into paper. In so many ways, Thay helps us know that in all forms of life—if we really look— we can trace the nourishing interconnectedness of our world.

A switch of perspective like this takes a little time. It also takes a commitment from you—a self-training as vital as any other.

To deal with your body's automatic responses to fear or to an impending disaster situation—which is how your brain is processing it— your top resource is to practice mindful conscious breathing. Or the whole-self breathing I offer in this book. Why? Because this tells your body there is no need for the stress responses that include rapid high breathing. *Bringing breath deep into your being grounds you, soothes and stabilizes you.* (There are so many apps that could guide you. I love to listen to chants also, ancient comforts that work just as well in our world today.)

Take time each day just to be present to yourself, and to something within or around you that restores aliveness and (relative) calm. This need not be formal meditation. It could be giving yourself completely to a piece of beautiful music. Or creating your own version of a tea ceremony—choosing your cup, choosing the tea, making it in a pot, sitting to drink it and feeling its warmth and familiarity as a grace.

As *Psychology Today*'s John A. Call says, "Be confident in your ability to deal with the tough stuff!" From Call comes this support, too, creating a "safety net" of preparedness. "Practice deep, even, controlled breathing when you aren't scared, and you'll be prepared to breathe this way when you do feel scared. Slow, even breathing helps to slow down your heart rate and lower your emotional arousal level." Anxiety, and especially panic attacks or terrors, inevitably rob you of control. (Any problems with breathing will do the same, including asthma attacks if you are unprepared and unmedicated.) *You reduce both anxiety (or fear) and stress when you can take at least some control of the situation, using your own body and breath to achieve that.*

Call also speaks up for meditation. I would urge you simply to think of this as being willing to notice and *rest* in the moment, rather than your body being in one place and your mind somewhere else.

Call writes, "Studies show that people who meditate daily have a thicker brain tissue in the prefrontal cortex, which is a part of the brain that handles working *memory, attention, and emotion regulation* [my italics]."

That's yet another benefit no one else can give you, *but you can claim for yourself.*

25 | Rehearse for "instant calm"

Is there any such thing as "instant calm"? Most people with anxiety will know too well how possible "instant panic" is, even when it's not a full-blown, confidence-shattering panic *attack*. But instant *calm*?

I, too, am wondering if "instant calm" is accessible in a hectic, overcommitted, or stressed life. In fact, it seems far safer to assume that *you may need to have some positive experiences of restoring calm well before overwhelming or confronting moments.*

During those most anxious moments, you are "flooded" inwardly. If you are ill, in severe pain, or suffering severe anxiety and depression, you can't easily access your most advanced organizing, initiating, calming-you-down faculties.

This is *not your fault.* Your body is doing what it should. *What it should not have to do is be on high alert much or most of the time.*

This is where even the simplest understanding of brain and body functions gives you precious knowledge of what is happening "out of sight" yet causing such disruption.

This is not to downplay the psychological, relationship, or inter-personal factors, and many social ones also pressing in on you. Nonetheless, deeper self-understanding means you can prepare for those dreaded moments, strengthening yourself—and causing your relationships and yourself least possible harm.

Calm breathing turns on the parasympathetic nervous system that tells your brain you are safe. Deeper breathing than usual brings more oxygen to the brain and lowers your levels of cortisol and other stress hormones.

Breathing is surely the most natural thing in the world. You breathe to live.

So, enjoy the tender care you give yourself when your breathing processes are turning "down" anxiety and turning "up" calm.

"Instant calm" requires some training, as anything does that's more complex than "instant coffee" or "instant noodles." (Even there, you need to have access to a power outlet and kettle.) *In fact, instant calm may be more accessible than coffee or noodles; with positive intention and a habit of practice, you can "have" it, at any time and in any place.*

You are never not breathing—until this life is over. How you breathe, however, varies with changes in and to your state of mind.

When you are very anxious, your breathing may become lighter, faster, in and out in the upper body. [That doesn't apply to my old friend, 3 a.m. worrying. Or to catastrophizing, or OCD (obsessive-compulsive disorder). Then, while the changes may be more subtle, they can still be addressed. Or rather, consciously breathing more slowly and deeply can in those situations also be calming.]

Human beings are creatures of habit, as most species are. Humans, though, have unique choices—including the choice to create new, conscious habits that benefit them.

Rehearsing for "instant calm" may be one of the most effective changes you can make. It is self-care at its best—because no one can do it for you; you can only do it for yourself.

The way to breathe more calmly involves breathing slowly and, with more attention, into your diaphragm, or belly, or whole self. Each time you breathe more slowly and into your whole being, you can use a conscious resolve in a single, tiny phrase. *Breathing slowly, I benefit myself. Breathing calmly, I benefit others.*

Calming breathing brings together what feels scattered within you. From feeling "all over the place," you begin to feel more centered and therefore more secure. Those are massive benefits. Like meditation, consciously slowed breathing can help us meet a hyper-anxious world with more detachment and exist more peacefully within it.

Never discount the simplicity of counting your breaths: ONE (counting ONE both in and out), TWO (counting TWO both in and out), and so on until TEN (counting TEN both in and out), before starting again. The more familiar this is, the more effortless, even "instant," it will be *when you really need it*.

The most valuable benefit of conscious breathing that I have found is that while it distracts then calms you, it also brings a little distance *within you* from anything that may be troubling you. (For some, repeating a familiar, trusted prayer can work just as well.)

That "little distance" becomes an opportunity for resting your mind, rather than being too "caught up." Each time you practice, you are taking effective care of your whole self. You are also caring for the social world you move and live in.

Part Three

Putting anxiety in its place

26 | Panic attacks are not all in the mind

What an amazing species we are! We have evolved over not millions but billions of years. And we continue to adapt to demands that are, as you read this, so new we can barely understand them. Systems of the body-mind that include the physiological, the neurological, and the psychological all influence how you are feeling. Plus, there are other factors that are more difficult to quantify, like the intrinsic value you are giving to your existence.

Over my lifetime, changes in how we understand anxiety have been profound. It's not the brain only that's shown to be "plastic" and able to heal itself in ways never before imagined. It is also the mind. Yet if anxiety is really troubling you, you might have said, or thought, "I would so much prefer to have something wrong with me physically that's easier to explain, if only to avoid other people's moral judgments that only seem to apply to feeling undone emotionally, never to a heart attack or cancer."

No matter how reluctant you may be to engage with
the "biology of anxiety," it helps to know that whatever
you are suffering is not "just in your mind."

Every part of you is involved; every part of you is affected.

You can, though, *enlist your mind to support you effectively.* Three ways
of doing this are vital. The first is to understand at least something about
the origins of panic in your life. This will help you to avoid situations
that might be triggering. It may also help you to find "grown-up" ways
of thinking about them, understanding that when you are in a panic,
your "thinking brain" is largely off duty.

I had the experience very recently of talking to a warm, very funny
woman in her forties, a computer engineer named Colette. She was
interested in talking to me about this book, but when I asked, gently,
about the nature of her panic attacks, her eyes almost immediately
filled with tears. It clearly was not the time and place, and I was struck
by how instantly even the thought of panic "attacking" her made Colette extremely uncomfortable. (Therapy could help. But in her case, it
needs to be trauma-based to be effective.)

The second point I would emphasize yet again is that *reducing stress
in your life is vital.* That's because your vulnerability to "panic" will
always be worse when your general levels of stress have become too
high—and your stress hormone levels are soaring.

**A panic attack can feel like a life-or-death crisis. The "danger"
that provoked it may be an "associated fear," rather than a
"real-time" one. But the body brain cannot tell the difference.**

My third point follows this. Your "panic responses" are triggered by neurological processes and by powerful stress hormones, especially cortisol. This is a glucocorticoid hormone linked with and more powerful than the better-known fight/flight/freeze response. (A little bit of bad news among the good: High cortisol levels are not helped by caffeine or high-density exercise . . . and both contribute to us pushing ourselves hard, or extremely. In stark contrast, a walk in the park, a visit to the library, a bookstore, or an art gallery, or sitting with a friend drinking tea, may be calming as well as connecting, though that may be my bias showing!)

It can be a high to feel an adrenaline rush, produced by your adrenal glands. It can be addictive. *It may not be healthy.*

Cortisol is made by your adrenal glands—the endocrine glands on top of each of your kidneys that are part of a larger endocrine system vital to healthy functioning. Not only does cortisol help to maintain blood pressure, it also maintains immune function and the body's vital anti-inflammatory processes. It is an essential hormone that affects almost every organ and tissue in your body. It plays many important roles, including the regulation of how your body metabolizes proteins, carbs, and fats, and how your body regulates blood sugar.

Glucocorticoids are a type of steroid hormone. They also affect sleep-wake cycles. (Oh, do they ever!)

Sleep—easy, lovely, restorative sleep—is often the first casualty when your anxiety/stress/cortisol levels are awry. *Just when deep rest is most needed.*

Your cortisol levels should be lower in the evening as you prepare to rest, and higher in the morning when you get up to face your day.

Your experiences of anxiety are influenced by many factors, external and internal. *Giving yourself the best chance to deal with the stresses that are part of everyone's life supports a depth of positive change only you can make.* Where this is triggering any degree of trauma from the past or is putting you in a state of near-constant "alert," *please seek and find intelligent help.* Self-care is something that can only happen in the "present tense," aware of what's needed—and doing that. Thinking about "maybe," "one day," "when I feel like it" doesn't take seriously your power to care as no one else can. I'm here, cheering you on. But nothing replaces a careful, thoughtful audit of what is causing stress and distress in your life right now.

Any expression of acute anxiety needs to be understood in a social context. Writer Meghan O'Rourke states it clearly: "We live atomized, exhausted, late-capitalist lives, running from here to there, eyes on our phones." In *The Invisible Kingdom: Reimagining Chronic Illness*, O'Rourke looks closely at the effects of these pressures on the body as well as the mind, drawing readers' attention to the intricate inter-relatedness of people with our environment. She notes the rise in autoimmune diseases (and long COVID) and suggests that the "immune-deregulated body" is, in her words, "an embodiment of our porousness to one another and of all the ways the body can be affected by personal interactions . . . systemic racism, poverty, trauma, and more."

27 | Can you blame your parents?

"Only 30 to 40 percent of the risk [of an anxiety disorder] can be accounted for by heritability. Which means environment is really critical as well."

NED KALIN, EDITOR-IN-CHIEF, *American Journal of Psychiatry*

Would it be fair—and entirely reasonable—to blame your parents for how anxious you are? Was it the genes you inherited? Or the (inadequate) way they brought you up? Perhaps your mother made a fuss about everything—except what really mattered? Or maybe it was your father who suffered from high blood pressure and a tendency to explode? Maybe you had grandparents who could not name their dreads, but you took them in anyhow. Or one side of your family of origin strongly disliked the other side. There may have been an overt fear or scorn of people who are "not like us," or who genuinely posed a threat through racism, religious bigotry, or other forms of prejudice. Or was it a widespread feeling of not-belonging? Or fear of the world beyond the family's immediate circles, or four walls?

You may indeed have a genetic predisposition to heightened experiences of anxiety. But genes and even a highly fraught family culture will only ever be a part of the story. If you have siblings, take a side-ways look at them: even in the same family it would be extremely rare if two siblings were living and feeling alike.

Personality traits do play a part. These include perfectionism, ti-midity, a propensity to ruminate or catastrophize in full color. Or to be easily undermined by what you assume other people are think-ing. A heightened and sometimes crushing sense of responsibility also brings burdens that I personally know all too well.

Among anxiety's harshest effects are flashbacks to past trauma, bringing new dread about what the future might bring and of your own competence to manage disappointments and setbacks.

Where there are such patterns in a family, and despite Dr. Kalin's clear words above, it may be extremely persuasive to tell yourself that this is a family story you cannot escape.

A few thoughts.

- Temperament exists in an innate form from the beginning. Yours shows up around things like energy, emotional responsiveness, hu-mor (or its absence), playfulness, exuberance, or shyness. Those innate features will then be modified or conditioned by your upbringing and circumstances.

- A tendency to overthinking, disproportionate worrying, nega-tive ruminating, or obsessive pessimism is *only 30 percent inherited*. This leaves 70 percent for environmental factors—including those where you have some choice and control.

- Self-absorbed, narcissistic parents or carers who saw you only as a reflection of themselves, or who trained you to believe in an om-niscient God judging your every wrong move, or who led chaotic or addicted lives, will not have been able to give you a strong inner foundation of safety. Yet, there is hope.

Whatever influences live within you, you are the author—ultimately— of your own life. The more conscious you are of this, and of the changes you can make to reflect your values and sense of self, the safer and more solid you will feel inside. *No one can give you that.* You can, though, claim it for yourself.

28 | You are the parent

Anxious parents worry that they will make their children anxious. That's a given. And it's undeniable that *all* parents will support their children best by reducing stress—especially where that appears to be "impossible." *Chronically elevated stress hormones benefit no one.* They can affect infants *in utero*, including temperament and their neurobehavioral development. This is an excellent reason to make reducing anxiety as well as stress a number-one priority for each individual, as well as for whole-family well-being.

Looking for the cloud's silver lining, I can confidently say, though, that an anxious parent (or, ideally, a now less-anxious parent) will be better informed than many others of the impact of ongoing environmental and social conditioning on their children. You may in fact be better able to support an anxious child toward greater inner security than a parent for whom this is foreign or unexplored territory.

Social anxiety is something many parents fear when they see signs of it in a child. The extroverted, assertive child does seem to function better in an extroverted society where much is clamoring

for our attention. A child—perhaps your child—who is more intro-
verted is easily overlooked in a busy classroom. That is painful to
witness. Almost every parent wants their child to be popular, sought
after, noticed, and appreciated. It's easy to feel our own long-ago
wounds when we witness a child we love struggling to be noticed.
Or chosen.

Frances is a school librarian and the mother of two daughters. It is
her elder daughter, Rosie, she spoke to me about.

My eight-year-old daughter, Rosie, is already showing signs of having a generally high level of anxiety (which runs in her family). She is pretty shy around
new kids and finds it hard to integrate into groups. She will quite often isolate
herself instead of integrating herself at school. I am an introvert myself, and
I really love my downtime after a day of being "on" at work. Also, I definitely
prefer one-on-one friendships. In school I always had a best friend and then a
cast of supporting characters. My partner is similar, but definitely more social
and has a slightly wider group of friends.

At school Rosie is very happy having one best friend and isn't making a
wide friendship circle, though she knows everyone and they all like her a lot.
Yet she is anxious. And she is very reluctant to make new connections. I see
her as vulnerable with just the one "best friend."

I have given her so much reassurance that she's a great kid and heaps of
fun to play with. I have explicitly encouraged her to make friends, reciprocate
warm greetings, not let herself be left out, and so on. But she is still riddled
with a deep-felt anxiety about socializing.

She describes it as feeling "scared" when she thinks about having to find
someone else to play with. If someone else makes the first move, she's fine

with that, and is totally up for playing with them. It's just her approaching another kid to ask them to play that fills her with anxiety.

What Frances is describing will be familiar to readers of all ages. A warm, thoughtful child—as Rosie is—is nonetheless reluctant to assert herself, to make the first move, to risk a rebuff. This is a kind of self-consciousness that at any age makes risk difficult and the world a scarier place than it needs to be. For an eight-year-old with relatively little life experience, it is a genuine conflict between retreating (as her instincts and inclinations urge) or advancing (as her parents urge).

I strongly suspect that Rosie is less convinced than Frances that "she's lots of fun to play with." Or even that she wants to be. There's a discrepancy here between "social norms" and what's an instinctual norm for Rosie. Nonetheless, some experiences of resilience will benefit Rosie. And will help her through harder challenges as she gets older.

Trying to protect Rosie from any and every rebuff is not helpful. Nor is encouragement to be someone she's not. *Rosie should not be enabled to avoid what's uncomfortable.* That will make her anxieties worse as she builds up the fears in her mind, rather than exposing them to daylight. *Avoidance is to be avoided, at any age!*

Keeping change low-key and unalarming is essential, with the same focus on strengths and creativity that's everywhere in this book. That could include a role-play that makes gaining insight fun.

TRY THIS

Invite Rosie to bring to mind how she is with her sister, her dad, or when someone is especially silly or fun. Let her name what psychosynthesis calls that "sub-personality," ideally with something to make her laugh, like Miss Peacock (who's not afraid to show her feathers). Then ask Rosie to give a loving, complimentary name to the part of her that is thoughtful and quiet, maybe something like Marvelous Hermione. Rosie could also give a respectful name to the part that's scared to put herself forward. That could be something like Miss Owl-Who-Watches. Or just Miss O.

This playful exercise teaches Rosie that we are not the same in every situation. *We play different roles within a single self.* Perhaps when she's ready, Miss Peacock can step forward to take a bit more of a risk than Miss O ever would, or that MH might want to. Emphasize that this is an experiment, that even if it doesn't go well, it's not wasted, and that maybe she could summon up an inner hero figure if she really wants to be daring. (And assure her that you, the parent, are going to try some play-acting experiments of your own.)

As all of us bumble along doing our best, take heart, too, from wise American writer Adele Faber, coauthor (with Elaine Mazlish) of the timeless book *Liberated Parents, Liberated Children.* She says, "I was a wonderful parent before I had children. I was an expert on why everyone else was having problems with theirs. Then I had three of my own."

29 | Conflict is always stressful

A great deal of anxiety—even anguish—comes when our personal relationships are not going well. Maybe it's hard to understand what's not working. Or why each person feels misheard and misunderstood, no matter how much talking there is. Or why there's so much fury? Or why attempts to clarify things make them worse?

Each person likely feels hurt. And defensive, which makes listening harder as anxiety, frustration, and hurt all grow. (Also, *louder* never helps.)

**Know that when you are already feeling anxious, you
will be especially sensitive to anything that you can
interpret as yet another blow to your shaky sense of self.**
You will be interpreting through a prism of hurt.
**Check whether you can step back inwardly and
look at any painful situation through a more
spacious, *more encouraging, whole-self perspective.***

There are many ways that you or I could view and interpret almost any situation—and make an internal story out of it. *Conflict is fired up by a difference in story.* That doesn't mean only one person or group is right. That kind of binary thinking entrenches conflict and doesn't relieve it. Much better to take it for granted that where there is conflict, there is hurt. Where there is hurt, there is defensiveness. Where there is defensiveness, it becomes harder still to guess at someone else's intentions and motivation. *It becomes all too easy to suspect and convince yourself of the worst.* And to become the tiger defending your territory.

Human consciousness means that we are primed to see "stories" through the prism of our cultural and social conditioning. Plus, those inner longings and yearnings that can be stronger than desires. It's also very hard to see past our inner defensiveness and long-held beliefs about how things "should" be. Or what someone else "ought" to be doing. Those are all conditioned expectations, sometimes barely conscious, that add outrage to anxiety. It's a potent mix.

It is truly liberating to understand that in any painful conflict situation unchecked assumptions will be flying. *Conflict is itself stressful.* (I cannot emphasize that enough.) *That makes it urgent to experience for yourself how possible it is to allow for interpretations that are more open and empathic than those that may first occur to you.* This "saves" you from worsening stress and anxiety, as much as it does anyone else.

That's especially true if you are already feeling defensive or hurt, vulnerable, and in any way under siege. Interpretations are key to how we tell stories and also hear them. Lots of novel reading helps! So does watching the best movies or series where at least some protagonists are capable of seeing events more clearly and consciously scene by scene, always with some setbacks.

Most of us believe that our interpretations are rock
solid. And they may be. Or maybe they represent
just one way of seeing things among many possibilities.

Understanding the stories that most affect you—
and looking at them freshly—brings a new sense of
connection. As well as the magic of empathy.

*Understanding and empathy can radically decrease anxiety and the distress
that comes with it.* They may even change your mood for the better—
and deepen those connections that really do matter to you. An example will make this clearer. (This example is one of so many I could
bring you because we live in a massively stressful, conflict-ridden society. Of course, effects of this will come "home.")

Paddy is a friend in our neighborhood, a devoted father in his
late thirties who suffers from dreaded panic attacks, mostly around
his work performance, even though his partner, Autumn, is (in her
words) "spending half my life reassuring him."

They have a baby girl together, Megan. Paddy also has a daughter,
Eliza, from a previous relationship. Eliza spends at least half the week
with them and, at fourteen, doesn't hesitate to inform Autumn she has
no right to tell her what to do, and there's no way she's going to "follow orders" from someone she "hates."

Autumn is feeling more insecure than she ever has. Megan is so
wanted, but Autumn had no idea how frazzled she would feel when
nothing about her routines is predictable. Perhaps she would be coping
better with her precious baby if she didn't feel undermined by Eliza's
cruel outbursts, and increasingly irritated by Paddy and his insecurity
dramas she now regards as unnecessary.

There is nothing here that is drastic. Yet no one feels good (except perhaps baby Megan). Each person feels poorly understood, vulnerable, and unacknowledged. Paddy can see that. What he can see less easily is how those big emotions are making it much harder for the adults to find workable strategies that would support them all. Meanwhile, Eliza—who believes she's almost an adult—is shouting like a three-year-old, and won't be free to access the full functions of her "thinking brain" for the best part of another decade. Eliza is stuck with black-and-white thinking, leaping from one extreme to another. Paddy and Autumn are not doing much better.

This is a situation that could quickly deteriorate further without insight. And with resentment building, rather than empathy.

Paddy, Autumn, and Eliza will be helped if they see and acknowledge that *each of them* is stressed and highly anxious as well as hurt. And while the stress for the new mother, Autumn, is especially great, physically as well as emotionally, that doesn't mean Paddy's or Eliza's feelings can be discounted.

I can only guess that there are other factors at work here that may be less conscious. For example, Paddy desperately wants his relationship with Autumn to flourish. He knows that with Eliza's mom, things went downhill fairly badly after Eliza's second birthday. He also knows that the family is experiencing financial stress with Autumn taking a year off from her work as a landscaper, while his work feels increasingly precarious. In his field of marketing, the rising stars are a decade or more younger than he is and are eager to work 24/7 with little or no time for a homelife.

In any of us, feelings of inadequacy quickly translate to feeling shamed—or angry. That makes everything harder. It's the "emotional brain" that's in overdrive here, creating stories of hurt and unfairness, plus fears that add up to "Who is taking care of me?" that can't possibly be articulated.

Goodwill is a magnificent asset, in my experience. It implies choice. It means never deliberately hurting another person. Wanting *the best for others.* Thinking of them warmly and kindly—and tolerating their usual human complexities.

> **Goodwill is an intention that clarifies insight as each person begins to step back a little from their own feelings, in an attempt to understand the others.**

Eliza, for example, is behaving badly toward Autumn when this is the last thing either of them need. Yet her strongest feelings are more likely about Paddy and Megan, not Autumn. Eliza is not jealous of the baby, but she is feeling stressed by school and fragile and reactive now because unconsciously she doesn't know how Megan's birth will affect her relationship with her dad, nor how they will regroup as a family of four, not three. Yet no one ever asks her how she is feeling—or that's her impression.

Autumn's vulnerability has been increased by giving birth to Megan, and by giving up her financial independence for a year, knowing that Paddy is never entirely comfortable with his work situation, on which they now all depend.

In a painful family drama like this one, a lot goes unspoken. Assumptions are made but not checked. It would always be ideal to have a counselor or wise friend to help each person listen to themselves, plus the others in turn. What is also immensely supportive is to have at least a broad-brush understanding of how emotions and emotional conditioning as well as values create "stories"—and where those "stories" could shift toward a more generous and empathic understanding.

This will make things less personal, and far less "hot."

Empathy creates relationship magic. It supports healing, not harming, inner narratives. It eases anxiety. It releases tension.

It says, "We want to understand one another. You are not alone."

Where each person can freely express their appreciation, and honestly and frankly say that *they feel in a muddle but have no intention of causing or sustaining hurt*, then the occasional outburst, snap, or adolescent rudeness can be better tolerated. The foundations of care can be trusted.

If there is a more effective way to ease relationship stress, I have yet to discover it.

30 | The power of memory

While our brains are terrible at remembering what is boring and familiar, they are phenomenal at remembering what is meaningful, what is emotional, and what surprises us.

LISA GENOVA

Your *Who am I?* sense of self is, to a surprising extent, made of memories, even the memories you are making right now as you read these words with some hope, interest, cynicism (which is it?). And where are you, as you read? What's around you, physically? What have you just eaten, or are you hungry? Are you fitting in some reading between other demands? How would you reply if I could ask, "What matters to you today?"

Most of that will seem so ordinary it's passing you by. "One day is much like another" may be your mantra. Yet no two days are exactly alike. You are not the same each and every day! Nor is your sense of self that will be shaped most by memories where you paid intense attention or felt something strongly—for better or worse. (If your mind is in a different place from your body, you won't easily remember where you parked your car, left your glasses, the name of a new person, or what you meant to buy at the supermarket.)

Intense memories are stored throughout your brain, but differently. Any somatic therapist knows they are also stored in your body, where trauma is certainly registered. Difficult, traumatic, or painful memories affect your hormonal systems, including those stress hormones like cortisol that register stress, causing you to panic, lose your breath, your heart to race. Or you sense danger, even when the actual or perceived danger was in the past.

Perhaps your partner or close friend is behaving callously. Trampling all over your vulnerabilities. Or someone you love is using again when they said they never would. Or you are about to be overlooked at work, again—or made redundant while other less hardworking employees are staying on. Or maybe yet another friend being "too busy" to make time to see you has tipped you into desolate loneliness. Or you have tried online dating and been rejected each time.

You feel the misery of that. You feel how powerless you are. And your unconscious mind creates an association between this "now" experience with other earlier crushing, defeating times. This causes additional anguish. *It also creates a feeling of continuity only with what has gone wrong, not with the other many, many experiences that have been more rewarding.*

An example came to me from a strong, intelligent woman I will call Annie. She's the mother of teenage sons, works in crisis management in a global company, yet feels trapped in conflicts with her own ex-husband, plus the opinionated, intrusive ex-wife of the man who is now her partner.

Both exes have poor boundaries. Annie is, in her own description, "somewhat anxious, though usually I manage it well."

Those experiences of being criticized, judged, even harassed from two directions over several years have, however, felt intolerable. As they would for any of us.

This is made worse because of the inescapable memories Annie has of being verbally abused and treated disrespectfully and hurtfully in her fourteen-year marriage. When her partner's ex is also joining in the criticism chorus—without knowing much at all about her or her circumstances—Annie finds herself veering between despairing misery and debilitating anger at the unfairness of it all.

I'm sharing this example (with Annie's permission) to demonstrate how acutely painful memories can bring the past into the present. This makes it essential to do some disentangling so that *other people's neuroses and/or projections—or their cruelty—will have less power to affect you.*

Do you wish that you could forget some of what you remember?

Do you wish that you could remember some of what you have forgotten?

Do you find old hurts rearing up when new hurts occur?

Or new hurts feeling more intense than makes "sense"?

Some of your anxious pain in the present moment is likely intensified by selective memories from the past that color your present reactions, jump-starting anxiety repeatedly. *That deserves your most compassionate, self-supporting attention.*

An understanding of memories and memory-making is surprisingly helpful. It can bring a new confidence to how you feel about yourself. It can diminish the understandable hurt you feel when other people are behaving in ways that throw you off-balance and seriously affect your peace of mind.

Even from a rocky start, it is possible to notice—take in, respond to—whatever stirs your curiosity, sense of beauty and sense of fun, and helps you to feel "more like yourself."

Those become great memories to talk about, intensify, and replay.

For Annie, some relief came from understanding it is the most emotion-drenched memories that get triggered, and *how* paying ever-closer attention to them by going over and over them in her mind gives both her partner's ex and particularly her own ex-husband far too much power to diminish and hurt her.

However difficult it first seemed, she had to *step back inwardly*, let some of their arrows fly by, see them as, yes, affecting her, but also part of *their* destructive patterns of relating, that she no longer needs to identify with and can and will detach from.

TRY THIS

If you are struggling with tension and anxiety (or anger) caused by fresh hurts and fears, check how "inevitably" your mind brings up memories of old hurts, *making the present moment even harder to bear.*

When you are able to look at a strong memory in a calm frame of mind, you reduce its power and perhaps release some of the anguish associated with it.

If you know that past memories are pressing in on your present life, notice which *patterns of memories* your mind is intensifying. Where this pattern is seriously affecting your mood, *seek intelligent professional help*— in addition to the changes you yourself can make. Your responses to the same memories are not static. They can change as you become less anxious, more inwardly stable, more conscious of their effect, and more in charge of where memory and thinking are taking you.

31 | The dopamine dilemma

I've found myself at one in the morning just sitting at
my desk spending an hour returning emails from the day
until like two in the morning. It's ridiculous. I should
be sleeping, or dreaming, or reading a novel.

BRIT MARLING

Focus is a frequent casualty when anxiety settles in long term. You may feel distracted and "all over the place." The multiple distractions of screens, myths around the virtues of multitasking, and being "on call" 24/7, don't help you, either. Your memory may be already adversely affected by anxiety or stress, along with your ability to initiate and organize. And while your attention may still be drawn back repeatedly to *what's wrong*, and what feeds rather than decreases your anxiety, your capacity to strategize or prioritize may also be under siege.

Waking up your power to sharpen your focus—and to exercise considerably more choice about *what you will focus on*—is self-therapy at its best. There are sound physiological reasons to do this, as well as psychological ones. Just as stress hormones like cortisol can drain or agitate you, the anticipation and planning of something positive or rewarding activates the release of dopamine in your brain.

This neurotransmitter—which acts in conjunction with serotonin and adrenaline as well as other hormones, plus glutamate—plays a vital role in many functions outside your conscious control, lifting your mood and potentially helping you with motivation, sociability, as well as paying attention. (Have you noticed that sometimes planning and getting ready for a big event is almost "bigger" than the event itself? Maybe wedding planners don't know this consciously, but they and their clients certainly live it out!)

However, while restoring pleasure is as vital for people suffering anxiety as it is for those robbed of pleasure by depression, high levels of dopamine, or overstimulation of the "reward functions" for short-term or even self-harming "rewards" tell a different story.

The dopamine dilemma is itself far from straightforward. Actor, writer, and producer Brit Marling speaks for millions when she says, "I used to be able to sit in a chair and for four hours straight in a very focused meditative way be in my own world without any interruption. And now it's like your brain is getting so trained to check your phone, and there is like a dopamine release every time you get a text, whether it's a good or a bad one. I'm really worried about what it's doing to our minds."

Seeking pleasure, seeking rewards, are states of mind we share with most species. One of the most precious things about human consciousness (and conscience), however, is that relative maturity lets us willingly defer short-term rewards, unless we are addicted (including addicted to our screens), in order to go for a bigger view of our own and others' needs, or for a longer-term or more widely shared benefit. More crucially still, consciousness and self-responsibility let us do something *because it is the right thing to do,* and not just for the pat and biscuit a puppy needs.

But the pursuit of pleasure for its own sake—and not as the *outcome* of a positive action or connection, or the drive for a dopamine rush—is seldom the kind of distraction that relieves anxiety and all that comes with it.

Very high levels of dopamine, perhaps unsurprisingly, can take you beyond reward toward delusions, mania, and hallucinations—not generally associated directly with anxiety but certainly with common forms of mood disorders. Hormones play a part here, too, affecting dopamine levels. *(This is most definitely psychiatry's territory, and if you suffer any of those effects, medical help is urgently needed.)*

Anhedonia is a loaded word that describes the loss of pleasure associated with depression. It's hard to endure. It is also near-impossible to imagine even for a clinician if you have not endured it. An absence of energy and motivation as well as pleasure, feeling helpless, and a detachment from things that once interested you are all familiar experiences for people with chronic and acute anxiety (and depression). They may express dopamine *deficiency*, perhaps worsened by a lack of sleep, a problem that inescapably seems to harm every aspect of our being.

At the time I am writing, there is not a simple medical test for dopamine levels to determine "too high, too low, or just right." What you can offer yourself, though, and the people who love you, is greater discernment around your activities, *noticing what drives the behaviors that have become most habitual,* then making self-caring, self-healing decisions as to what you will pursue. And what you will not.

Patience is often another casualty, both of anxiety and these arguably dopamine-fueled times. Agitation and overstimulation are the enemies of patience and the resilience, tolerance, and calm that come with it.

Is it possible to reinstate patience in your life? Writing in his short book *Dopamine Detox,* author Thibaut Meurisse points out, "Watching motivational videos all day long won't help you reach your goals. But, performing daily consistent actions, sustained over a long period of time, will [help you reach your goals]. Staying calm and focusing on the one task in front of you every day [also] will."

Choosing where your attention goes, and where that attentiveness is taking you, may need some practice. This is basic mindfulness. Or self-awareness leading to conscious choices. You can, for example, choose *to look out for what's going at least half well:* where someone did in fact say something kind or funny, when the food you cooked and ate did taste pretty good, when an unexpected insight rose up in the privacy of your own mind, or when a part of your body is *not* aching or disappointing right now. Psychologically or physiologically, unless you are catastrophically "flooded," human consciousness almost always gives you some degree of choice.

The Japanese therapy called Morita offers you something useful here. I have always been fascinated by how Morita philosophy prioritizes *well-chosen action* over emotion-driven decision making. ("I don't feel like it" can be a tyranny. Dependent behaviors are also a trap.)

Morita therapy suggests *acknowledging whatever your feelings are,* rather than attempting to shift or ignore them, yet rather than being ruled by those feelings, choosing to *do something because it needs to be done.* Or because it can make a positive difference.

Action can shift feelings, not least because your focus has shifted. And even if your feelings don't change, you have still done what needs doing. *You have moved forward,* favoring your power to choose over habits of anxiety. And over whatever infinitely complex interactions of hormones and neurotransmitters with conditioned emotions and responses might otherwise hold you back.

A final note: if you have an ADHD (attention deficit hyperactivity disorder) diagnosis, you might think you should be in the front line for a dopamine detox, but this is very much a matter to work on with a treating psychiatrist because "due to [a] lack of dopamine, people with ADHD are 'chemically wired' to seek more," says John Ratey, associate clinical professor of psychiatry at Harvard Medical School and coauthor, appropriately, of the book *Driven to Distraction.*

32 | My name is also not Anxious

No person can ever decide what another
person needs to learn and needs to do.
ANNE WILSON SCHAEF

Appearances tell a partly truthful story. A quick glance at me and you
would likely see that I am positive, creative, curious, and, I hope, caring. And that's correct. I have a greatly loved and loving family, and
dear friends with whom I can be "myself." My professional life has
been varied, challenging and more adventurous than I could ever have
imagined as a convent schoolgirl in New Zealand.

I can get up in public and speak to a thousand people if I am well
enough prepared. I can work in a fiercely competitive field (writing)
without feeling overly daunted. But my boldness has limits. As yours
might have.

For much of my life I have lived with some degree of anxiety. As
a child, I had vivid and frightening nightmares—a few of which I
can recall decades later. I didn't hear anyone name fearful repetitive
thoughts as obsessional. Yet I felt their power. I was easily terrified by

150

other people's stories of horror, ghosts, or "bad things happening." Like you again, perhaps, I have been fully awake at 3 a.m. and unable to go back to sleep far more often than I care to remember.

Insomnia, stress, and anxiety make an unholy trinity: one of them is seldom present without the other two. *A vivid imagination hasn't always been my ally.*

Anxiety is not something that can be fully understood by observing it, reading about it, or studying it. I know that. Nor can its pervasiveness be understood by someone who feels "het up" from time to time or experiences "butterflies" or "nerves" or a wakeful night before a big occasion. That can be uncomfortable. But chronic or severe anxiety is visceral. It lives in your guts as much as it does in your head. It can raise your temperature, make your heart race, cause you to panic, vomit, collapse. It can make you feel sick, hot, flushed, exhausted, heavy—anything but fully alive.

High levels of anxiety make clear thinking hard or impossible. Despite my apparent confidence as a child, I was in dread that something would happen to my mother. And it did. She died of cancer in her thirties when I was eight and my older sister only eleven. My inner stability was gone. So was my power to see myself through the eyes of unconditional acceptance and love, though I had no language for that.

It would take years of therapy as an adult, years of writing, thinking, and becoming a mother myself, to find a more reliable steadfastness within myself. I also had to discover that there is no "closure" for a fundamental grief. You grow around it. And while, yes, it may add to your compassion for others' suffering, it also makes your own inner world perilous, long before it should be.

Even now, decades after my mother became ill and died, if someone I love is seriously unwell, my fears can become overwhelming.
Easy sleep disappears—if I ever had it. I eat too much or too little. I go
into an unhealthy state of full alert and, unless I am careful, I will hear
inside my mind, "It's up to you to rescue . . . to do more . . . Perhaps
worrying more intensely or profoundly will 'do it,' whatever 'it' is.
Either way, you cannot relax for a minute."

Some of this overalertness, overanxiety may be genetic. Some of it
is learned. Fundamental issues of attachment and separation, belonging and abandonment, play out in many of us throughout a lifetime.

My paternal grandmother was abandoned as a child when first
one parent disappeared (in India?), and then the other. My maternal
grandmother outlived four of her seven adult children. She modeled
extraordinary grace and stoicism in her kindness to all her grandchil-
dren. My adored grandfather did also. Yet it was impossible to ask or
be asked, "How are you coping? What does it feel like to be you in
your utterly changed world?"

Despite profound intergenerational grief, no spoken language was
available for naming anyone's experiences. I read voraciously but found
no language in books, either, for the fears I felt through those childhood years, or the grief I dared not express—and shrank from, appalled,
when it was hinted at by others. I also had no language to comprehend
all the denial and self-medicating that was going on around me.

What I did know was that I hated the way that so many men of my
father's generation drank alcohol as though it was their sole comfort.
(Perhaps it was.) While women—who drank far less than men in those
days—were somehow "responsible" for the emotional well-being of
everyone around them. Again, without language. At the same time,

their strengths and fortitude were often trivialized, and their significant anxieties or legitimate frustrations ignored. (*Valley of the Dolls*—called "the best worst novel of all time" by the *New York Post*—was shocking because it dared to name its female characters' dependence on barbiturates.)

World events affected me, along with my personal, hidden griefs and fears. I was (justifiably) afraid of war, of nuclear threats, of state-sanctioned harm to women and children. I was proud of New Zealand for its antinuclear stance.

Where I was unafraid was in joining others in social activism and protesting. During the sixteen years I lived in Europe before coming to live in Australia, I protested wars, called out sexism, and denounced the entwined violence of racism and poverty. One of the most terrifying experiences of those years was when I sat, with who knows how many others, spread out across a main road in the South London suburb of Brixton. Our aim was to bring traffic to a halt and draw attention to a just cause. It was one of countless anti-racist protests but on this occasion the police came riding in on their huge horses. And kept coming, daring us to test our resolve against a very real prospect of being trampled. Such cowards.

In hyper-tense moments like that, the experience is more physical than emotional. Terror is a *felt* experience. But the emotional scars that fear leaves—or any trauma, including grief—fester as anxiety in its many forms. *The world feels less safe. I feel less safe.*

Today, like billions of others, I worry desperately for our threatened world as it warms and suffers. I worry for all those people who are dispossessed or experiencing extreme hardship, which a fairer, kinder world would not tolerate. I cannot watch violent movies or series, or read thrillers or any fiction that promises horror. I am particularly triggered by stories of children's sufferings.

Over a lifetime, as many as 40 percent of women and more than 25 percent of men are likely to experience anxiety that significantly affects their quality of life. And while statistics don't help in those wide-awake early hours, insight does.

With the support of therapy, self-therapy, insight, years of freeing, positive spiritual practice, and a kind of stubborn optimism born out of my belief in humankind's essential goodness—despite much evidence to the contrary—I have almost always been able to be busy, absorbed, sociable, and enthusiastic.

That's reflected in my books, friendships, parenting. I can now live more freely knowing myself better, knowing what our minds are capable of, and trusting my capacities to heal. Remaining hopeful seems to me to be the essential act of courage.

It is, too, an act of commitment to life itself.

33 | Body anxiety

*We weren't born into the world hating our
bodies. This is something society has taught us.
Body shaming is a universal problem.*

TARYN BRUMFITT

Body anxiety is something that blights far too many lives, along with
the multiple eating disorders that are on the rise. Numbers are little
consolation. Anxiety about your physical self—your one, precious,
mortal, vulnerable body—is a tragedy for each person experiencing it.
It is also a pain-filled example of how intensely and effectively we are
conditioned by the time, place, and culture we live in.

Bit by bit, judgment by judgment, one absurd media beat-up after
another, little children grow bigger, discovering as they grow what
their body shape, ethnicity, race, size, and skin color "ought to look
like" by grossly superficial standards. And also, what their appearance
might mean to critics. While there's little justice or basic sense to it,
virtually no one escapes scrutiny, plus narrow-minded, stereotyping
judgments. And *virtually no one escapes confusing their physical self with far
deeper issues of identity.* Character, values, ethics, creativity, kindness,

155

and brilliance can be completely disregarded when the all-important "looks" triumph in the judgment stakes.

> **The real tragedy is that when you live with anxiety about how your body is perceived and judged, your "whole self" feels at risk. Confusing "me" with "my appearance" is all too easy when "appearance" is frequently registered first, second, and last.**

Racism and sexism are wicked tools in the body-shaming kit. So, in the West, is ageism, with some women in their fifties, sixties, seventies, or older struggling, starving, and/or submitting to surgery to try to look eternally thirty-five. This is more than an issue of sexual desirability. It also relates to a reluctance to accept the unavoidable truths of our mortality. ("As long as I look thirty-five, or forty-five, I can avoid the realities of old age, illness, and death. Perhaps I would rather experience body anxiety, now in the present, than face my anxiety about death.")

I thought I knew a good deal about this issue, yet I was shocked and saddened to learn that almost 90 percent of adult women in Western cultures have body acceptance challenges, plus increasing numbers of men. Children, too, report it as one of their major concerns—not how healthy, strong, vigorous, or adventurous they are, but how rigidly they conform to norms *decided by other people*, many of whom profit to an eye-watering extent from exactly these anxious obsessions.

The superficiality of these judgments, and how successfully they are exploited for profit, shows up in the multiple ways that we are trained—yes, *trained*—to pay far more attention to appearances than to what kind of people we and others are. It's far easier, and certainly far more commercially rewarding, to obsess about someone's weight, skin color, age than their values, character, loyalty, kindness. Or how interested as well as interesting they are.

This focus matches that of contemporary society as a whole. Advertising, media, and commercial "interests" dominate how you create your perceptions—even your innermost perceptions of yourself. "I hate my body . . ." is a tragic, learned response. In too many lives, this can lead to body dysmorphia and eating disorders. Globally, the lifetime prevalence of eating disorders is around 8.4 percent for women and 2.2 percent for men. These disorders are serious mental illnesses and are life-threatening if untreated. Cultural influences are integral to this picture.

Insight, however, tells you that unless you are seriously unwell you have choices around perceptions and attitudes, including *how you feel about yourself.* These external, often toxic cultural influences can be seen for what they are. They are exploiting your anxieties about not fitting in, about not being loved, desirable, wanted . . . not being in some crucial way "enough."

Actor and writer Hannah Vanderheide has written, "I'm an eating disorder survivor with two autoimmune diseases that both cause rapid weight loss during flare-ups. And while I may be only a single case study, I'm representative of just a few of the many reasons why weight *gain* is, quite often, something to be celebrated. *When my body drops weight, it's because I'm sick. When it's bigger, I'm well* [my italics]."

Rebellion is called for. Why should the commercially self-interested decide how you should look? Or feel? Do they know you? Do they care about you and your well-being? Or that of your loved ones? I'd say not. Compassionate, self-respecting insight restores your sense of what matters most (your health and emotional as well as physical well-being, not *other people's judgments*). Insight lets you choose to cherish rather than condemn your body, to appreciate rather than scorn it. ("My body is okay, but I hate looking old / effeminate / too heavy / too dark / too light / too fat / not tall enough / too tall / plain / ugly . . .")

> **You can choose to honor your body's genetic and cultural story—and care for it. This can and will positively influence every aspect of your being.**
>
> **You can treasure everything about your body's miraculous ability to heal and survive; to learn and change; to feel pleasure and offer kindness.**
>
> **You can honor—and appreciate out loud—your own and others' heroic efforts to live well with chronic pain or disability. Or the effects of sexism, racism, poverty. You can celebrate any step away from the conformity that might suit a billion others, but not you.**
>
> **You can bring greater sense to your own body—and to the "body" of our world.**

Anxiety about your body's appearance is not "natural." It is not inevitable. You can look at it—and yourself—through fresh eyes. You can become clear about how body anxiety or body-shaming are causing you harm. Or worse. You can also decide whether this is how you want to live. Gaining fresh insights about your perceptions and attitudes, and changing them to be self-healing, is the basic premise of this book. Where you are harming yourself with your own self-criticism or even self-hatred, *that can be changed.*

This is the nub of self-acceptance: to make peace with your body, to understand it and your whole self well beyond "appearances," to accept and care for it, to be grateful for all your body's efforts, to know that *while you are more than a body, you and your body are one.*

TRY THIS
Many people are *their own harshest body shamers.* Start there. You may not be able to stop other people judging you or anyone else in superficial, banal ways. You *can* stop yourself. You can establish your own values. You can live by those, rather than the values of the crass, exploitative commercial worlds and media.

- *Ruthlessly ban all self-hating phrases from your vocabulary.* No matter how loud those internal voices of self-denigration are, or how pervasive your envy of those (improbably) "perfect others" may be, silence them. See them as a product of materialistic systems that damage your relationship to yourself. Also, ban all disparaging, stereotyping words from your comments about other people. Whatever their age, culture, or race, they share your desire to belong and be appreciated.

- *Consciously identify small gestures of wellness and strength*, and especially what you might not always be able to take for granted. After four or five years of injury, I still cannot lift the newest baby in our family. But I can hold her on my knees and in my arms. I can bend down to pick something up off the floor, I can walk to the shops and back. I can sit in my chair and type these words on my laptop. Hurrah!

- *Notice what you most appreciate about other people.* Where it is generous and healthy, use that as your prism through which to view them. Contribute to a world that values good humor, character, generosity—and kindness.

• *Speak aloud your appreciation of other people—not "just" their appearance.* Comment lavishly on their heartwarming, uplifting, and generous characteristics. Be grateful they are in your life, and you in theirs.

To live in a state of harmony with your own body is as essential to self-care as anything could be. Mind and body are not separate, as I so often remark here. But nor is that essence we might call spirit, soul, or life force—vibrant in a whole-self picture. As I've written in the past, "Your attitude to life is far more important in determining your happiness than your money, appearance, social status, or talent." Choosing a positive attitude toward your physical "self"—and your unique gift of life—is central to your well-being.

34 | What happened to you?

Amazing how by asking "What happened to you?" instead of "what's wrong with you?" you can shift the blame from the person experiencing mental health problems to the circumstances that contributed to their distress like trauma, abuse and poverty.

DR. AHMED HANKIR

Maybe anxiety has been hanging around in your life "forever." It's also possible that specific events or experiences have tipped you from "managing" to "not doing so well." Or worse. Dr. Hankir, whom I quote above, is known as "The Wounded Healer." That's a phrase taken from the early Swiss psychiatrist Carl Jung. It implies a welcome honesty: that those of us who work with others in their healing are simultaneously engaged in healing ourselves. It could not be otherwise in my experience.

Nor is it "professional" healers only who should be included. It's all of us willing to acknowledge our inescapable interdependence, as well as how much we can learn from others. In fact, I would go so far as to say that *all true healing relies on an I–Thou connection* of some kind that reaches beyond the mind and body to spirit and soul.

The phrase "I–Thou" is a profound one and relevant to the way you regard others or assume (or fear) how they view you. It was coined by Austrian-Jewish philosopher Martin Buber.

Buber contrasted the authentic acknowledging of the other person in any I-Thou connection with the dehumanizing experience of I-It where who you are is reduced to your functions, or use, and you are responded to accordingly. (Sacking someone by email would come into this category. So would breaking off a relationship using a text message. Or being dropped by an old friend as she becomes "important" and you do not. Or working in service industries or retail and being treated as though you have no existence but to do customers' bidding. Or being seen, as Ahmed was, as "worthless" because he was mentally ill, homeless, and suicidal. Or being known only by your diagnosis.)

Buber died in 1965 and, in the years since, perhaps made worse by social media, *people increasingly have felt unseen as individuals*, often while being judged against demeaning or unrealistic stereotypes.

Any experience where you are disrespected, or your essential humanity is ignored, affects your mental health. If you are particularly dependent on other people's reassurances of your worth, this will be even harder to bear.

Striving to see others as whole people, and letting others see you as a whole person, is what brings an I-Thou connection. Yet when it comes to mental health or its absence, it is still a comparatively rare psychiatrist who will come "out" as someone who was, in Ahmed's words, "hopeless and suicidal," as many of his patients and some readers of this book may be.

Stigma around mental illness remains life-threatening when people fear speaking out and avoid treatment for fear of "exposure." Any health system that sees anxiety or any other mood disorder as solely an individual "problem," or as something to be feared and hidden, itself has severe problems. *The social and cultural pressures on some of us are particularly acute. Pretending this is not happening helps no one.*

You also live in a deeply personal world. *Whatever happened to you* may be acutely, intimately harmful. No one survives a painful situation without some trauma. While it may not be diagnosable as PTSD (post-traumatic stress disorder), there will be triggers that attack your confidence and self-worth.

Adverse events, as the medical people call them, might produce more stress than you can tolerate. This can result in a breakdown of health that primarily affects the body, even while it threatens to break your heart or spirit. I believe this happened to me when I had breast cancer in my forties, at the same time as I was dealing with a particularly demoralizing (and unnecessary) family property dispute. I have since heard multiple similar stories. *Frightening events breed more fear . . . that is felt everywhere in your body.* They accelerate any degree of anxiety you already have. They make the world feel dangerous and can make you feel powerless.

Recognizing "what happened to me" won't be relevant for everyone. But it does open you to the reality that what you are feeling—and assuming—today may well be affected by circumstances of yesterday.

And that *underlying persistent as well as acute anxiety will continue to affect your whole self*: body as well as mind, emotions as well as spirit. And it is most effectively eased from the same perspective.

Ahmed was saved from destroying himself because his Islamic faith forbids suicide. "That's what deterred me," he says. Surviving this desperate experience has made him a fierce advocate for caring courageously and intelligently for our mental health, a message he has shared in nineteen countries.

We are all wounded. We are all healers. Recognizing that in one another creates an I-Thou truth almost greater than any other.

35 | The power of attitude

The power your attitudes have is revealed through actions and behaviors—and maybe most of all through those famed "Freudian slips" when you say what you didn't quite mean to . . . it just "slips" out. Those are telling moments. They can also be awkward ones. So it is worth consciously exploring what your driving attitudes may be: about yourself and your life, about other people and their power to influence you—as well as what you most value and care about.

Insight, again, lets you glimpse what's driving those "I didn't mean to" moments. It also supports you as you unravel the story of your emotional self, through which you take in events—and express your responses. That requires a challenging question or two, not least about you and anxiety.

How often do you think about whether—or how—your most fundamental attitudes are affecting you? Is this something you would like to understand better?

Are you conscious of how they are influencing what you aspire to (not only materially, but even more in the relationship realms)?

Finally, but not least, what are your attitudes toward anxiety, and toward the YOU who is sometimes or often troubled by the disruption anxiety brings to your inner confidence and harmony?

There are, please be assured, no "right" answers, nor any wrong ones. This is not about your ability to "think positively." *As a measure of future well-being, that is very much just one factor among many.* Access to first-rate care, your genes, financial security, your social support, unanticipated complications, and so much else besides, all play a major role.

Certainly, a positive attitude may make it easier to endure or cooperate with any medical treatment that is painful or arduous. (Some treatments for mental illness are every bit as hard to endure as those for physical disease.) But around this topic swirl many judgments, including the outrageously incorrect one that surviving a diagnosed terminal illness can be brought about through your serenity or positivity of mind. *It cannot.*

When it comes to mood disruptions—remembering that anxiety is the most treatable—questions of attitude become more interesting. And, I believe, more authentically hopeful. This is because the complex ingredients that make up "attitude" include unconscious as well as conscious factors. In the mix, too, are beliefs, opinions, reactiveness, conditioned thinking (what your culture, time, and place have trained you to assume), and—of course—the full range of your emotions.

Letting yourself see more clearly what your attitudes are—and whether they are supporting you, or not—brings abundant insight.

With insight comes choice to respond to your emotional distress and challenges with greater compassion and self-trust.

Two examples follow to bring this to life. The first addresses a common challenge for people who suffer confusion about what their priorities really are. And also, great anxiety about doing the "right thing" in the eyes of other people . . . while *frequently neglecting to do right by themselves or their loved ones.*

This is certainly a habit driven by deep attitudes that can be quite unconscious, especially that your "worth" in others' eyes is dependent on each individual performance, rather than holding on to a bigger picture of what you do and how you do it. Plus, a much bigger, kinder view of yourself.

Henry is a Christian minister of religion. He's immensely generous with his time and interest to his friends as well as his congregation. He is highly involved in a number of interfaith and multicultural events. He has energy to burn for others, but not for his partner, Tom. This is such a cliché of a story, yet as Tom says, "Living it is still an individual experience. I feel as if I have no right to demand more from Henry and any time I do raise it he veers between irritability or placating me, often saying he will do more around the house or we will take some time out together when, actually, what I want most are times that are not deep, not heart-to-heart, just lazy and companionable.

"Does his attitude toward himself and his Christian duties allow that? I am not at all sure. I thought of Henry as a free spirit for years. Now I see that he is as driven by duty as any twentieth-century clergyman but is just far less conscious about it—and therefore far less available to be challenged."

My second example is more familiar, and wonderfully domestic. I say "wonderfully," because it is in our hearts and homes that "attitude" is most truthfully revealed, especially when our attitudes contribute to our own or someone else's anxiety.

In *The Book of Overthinking*, popular author and psychologist Gwendoline Smith (aka "Dr. Know") urges eliminating the words "should," "must," and "have to," all of which have the potential to arouse resentment and pressure in anyone prone to anxiety.

Clever (wise) Dr. Know knows to make a clear distinction between "instructional shoulds" that usefully tell us what to do and how to do it, and "moralistic shoulds" that have their origins in other people's views, beliefs, and opinions, and can create tension, stress, anxiety, or illness in us.

There are, though, times when you may be imagining the "shoulds" and the "musts." You may be projecting your sense of obligation onto someone else, particularly when you are unsure about other people's expectations of you—how essential it is to keep winning their approval, plus your own confusion about what matters most.

Juggling expectations and priorities is difficult when you feel well.

When you feel anxious, it can be a hundred times harder. Speak to yourself like a friend. Or a kindness coach: "What would help?"

Confusion accompanies fear-driven thinking and needs cool checking. "Why must I? Who would I be letting down if I do—or do not—obey this 'must'? Where and how am I taking care of myself—or the people I am most responsible for? Where and how am I asking for help—and showing a willingness to accept it?"

Dr. Know points out, and I agree with her, "Instructional 'shoulds' are helpful . . . Fear-driven motivation makes people ill. True motivation comes from *the desire to do something* [my italics]."

Yes, there will be many times when you do something that simply needs doing. My earlier reference to Morita therapy (in chapter 31) suggests that this can be an excellent method to shift self-limiting feelings. You will get on with it. You will do it. No big deal. But in a self-encouraging, self-accepting life, where you are treating yourself *and* others with interest and respect, that means keeping alive your firsthand experience of choice.

Dr. Know gives an example. She writes, "Instead of thinking, *I should do all of the housework today, it has to be done and it must be done today*—which sounds like time for a cup of tea and a lie down with the raging headache you've just given yourself—try thinking this way: *I could do the housework today. But I've had a big week, so I might do some today and leave the rest for tomorrow.* Now, doesn't that feel better?"

36 | Other people's opinions

*We live today in an "age of anxiety" . . . The ordinary
stresses and strains of life in the changing world of today
are such that few if any escape the need to confront
anxiety and to deal with it in some manner.*

ROLLO MAY

A few years ago, I set out to write a book about my experiences of a
difficult combination of serious illnesses. Because writing is my way of
understanding things better, I thought putting what happened to and
within me onto the page might help me, and possibly others. It didn't.

I wrote almost half a book before I realized that I could not put
enough of myself into it to make it meaningful for others yet could
not put myself into it any more than I had without reliving trauma
that was still too acute. (My admiration for super-courageous books
like *When Breath Becomes Air* by Paul Kalanithi is profound.)

I also could not see how I could fill out my more philosophical
reflections on illness (mortality and death) with palatably funny, absurd, or touching personal anecdotes, or even particularly inspiring

170

ones. There may be sections I can revive at some point, particularly to reflect my gratitude to the loved ones who supported me, and sorrow for the many who have no one to sit with them when they are beyond words or lost for them. But a whole polished book? No.

The fact is that I wasn't well enough to be writing. That experience of coming up short showed me how we struggle to express ourselves adequately in the face of our own or soneone else's serious illness. How can *we* make sense of it, never mind those who are looking on? Yet I also experienced how eager many well-intentioned people are to share their opinions, even when their understanding of your situation is based only on their own subjective assumptions.

Anxiety can be more than an experience. It can be disabling, limiting, like any chronic or serious illness with acute patches. To recognize that *you are more than your anxiety*—and to take charge of your attitude toward yourself and life once more—is not simply a good idea worth trying. It can be life-changing.

Irish poet-philosopher Pádraig Ó Tuama writes in *Poetry Unbound*, "Anybody who has lived with chronic illness will know that not only must you learn to live with your own symptoms, but you must also learn to live with other people's opinions about your symptoms: whether your illness is valid or not; whether you should or shouldn't take this medication or that; what will help; what will not help; whether the illness is your fault; whether you're believed or not. This is a burden on top of your body's burdens. Living with people's readings—people's moral readings really—about your pain can make everything worse."

Chronic illness, including chronic anxiety or depression, can make other people particularly uncomfortable. (Many people are fine in a crisis; less so in the longer haul.) Yet they may still be quite intrusive in their views. Detach as best you can. Some of what people say that's most unwelcome reflects their own stress. Or fear of what has been particularly difficult in their own or loved ones' lives.

Totally ill-informed commentary cannot help you. You gain a little power when you decide it is not going to harm you, either.

Anxiety is affecting people of all ages in unprecedented numbers. I wonder that anyone's life remains untouched, directly or indirectly. Our very planet is "nervous," says a writer as influential as Britain's Matt Haig. Yet when it is YOU who is sleepless, agitated, insanely worried, checking and rechecking, facing the same thought with the regularity of tuna on the sushi train when you are a vegetarian . . . when any of those or a thousand things are happening that are getting you down and further down, is it any comfort to know you are one of millions? I don't think so.

When someone expresses an earnest opinion about your state of mind, they are making an uninformed guess. At best. They don't have a window to your inner world. They don't know—even if they are utterly committed to your well-being—what it is to be you. (In the hardest times, you may not know what it is to be you.) What you do know, though, is that some of the precious patience you feel for yourself will, by necessity, have to be shared around.

Taking tiny, necessary steps to tolerate other people's clumsiness with more ease, you may find yourself better able to tolerate your own.

Sowing the seeds of noticing, gathering in the harvest of insights, is both a collective and a very individual activity. Sometimes you will need saving from your own loneliness. Sometimes you will need to protect your own solitude.

"People" are you. Me. All of us. The wise and the very unwise. Protecting yourself from harm that comes from the "outside" is legitimate and urgent. Protecting yourself from harm that comes from the "inside" is vital and lifesaving.

Pádraig is so right to say, "Living with people's readings—people's moral readings really—about your pain can make everything worse." This is never truer than when it is a mental illness, a "disregulation" of mood, a "failure" to love life as you should.

None of us escapes the inner voice, also, that says, slyly, "Stand up a bit straighter. Think about someone other than yourself." Or, "What have you got to complain about with your comfortable life and a roof over your head?"

But people's "moral readings" may also and perversely make things better. They can remind you that *you are the leader and guide in your own healing.* That however flat you feel, your insights will have a depth that no one else's can rival. And maybe the truth is that their reading lets you know how far off the mark they are, and how close to the mark you are.

I'll give Matt Haig the last word. He writes in *Notes on a Nervous Planet*, "You don't put out a fire by ignoring the fire. You have to acknowledge the fire. You can't compulsively swallow or tweet or drink your way out of pain. There comes a point at which you have to face it. To face yourself. In a world of a million distractions, you are still left with only one mind."

37 | You are not a machine

Mistakes are at the very base of human thought, embedded there, feeding the structure like root nodules. If we were not provided with the knack of being wrong, we could never get anything useful done. We think our way along by choosing between right and wrong alternatives, and the wrong choices have to be made as frequently as the right ones. We get along in life this way. We are built to make mistakes, coded for error.

LEWIS THOMAS

I witnessed an impassioned conversation recently between two women, both of whom are medically qualified and both of whom have had their own struggles with debilitating forms of anxiety (one with a yearslong eating disorder, the other with panic attacks). They were discussing why, in addition to the very real social and environmental pressures of this time, anxiety seems to be more prevalent now than it was a generation ago.

Their conclusion was that because of social media many of us live our lives more publicly and competitively than ever before, while the pressures have grown greater to be seen to be doing well *in every sphere of life*. We are comparing ourselves, they suggested, to straw idols, images of achievement that intensify self-doubt and grossly undermine our necessary confidence that we will take ordinary experiences of "failure" or setbacks and disappointments in our stride.

In that same week, I saw on television a conversation with a university educator of preschool teachers who was making a confident case for preschoolers learning conceptual thinking. She explained its value with a strange example, so that instead of running up and down the aisles to discover where, for example, toothpaste is, they would know that toothpaste is a *category* that they could quickly find.

I found this discussion depressing. (I also find it worse than depressing that rote learning is increasingly tested in kindergarten via spelling lists, "homework," and inane readers for five-year-olds who could be listening to myths and legends, or dancing or chanting, playing make-believe and having creative *fun*.)

This emphasis on younger and younger children valuing just a constricted version of cognitive skills above all others seems to me a backward step. It has so little to do with creativity, the power of story, and living fully and vigorously in your own body, alongside others and in an awesome world.

With so much emphasis in later life on intellect and performance, and conflating that with a person's value, it would seem a rebellion is called for. Would we be less anxious, I can't help but ask, if we were to regard our own lives not as something to be whipped into shape, but as something *unfolding*, always with more to discover—whatever the inevitable bumps you will meet?

A fear of making mistakes plus a dread of *being seen to be wrong*, or just not being the mythical "best," is a catalyst for panic attacks for many, and grumbling anxiety for many more. Some of this comes from perfectionism (which I understand all too well), also from the way we internally construct a limited and often unrealistic image of *how we want to be seen.*

It's a cruel fallacy that people will love us more if we are "perfect" in every way or a "winner" every time. In fact, if such a person does exist, they will suffer others' very mixed feelings including envy, and possibly *schadenfreude* (a wry pleasure that someone is *not* doing so well) when they do show up as fully, wonderfully human.

It is profoundly freeing to accept yourself as someone who is most definitely not a machine (!), who is evolving in self-knowledge and in every other way, and *who can make inevitable mistakes and learn from them rather than obsessing about them.*

Recognize where your critical judgments of others—as well as of yourself—are limiting a depth of connection that can only come when *we accept one another in our complexity.* Not as that airbrushed version of self who appears to have it "all in hand," nor as someone who can "keep going," no matter what.

"Keeping going no matter what" is a contemporary badge of honor. I am susceptible to this—and there have been times when it combined well with my energy and drive. There have been plenty of other times, though, when I observed no warning signs whatsoever until I was ill. Or when I allowed my mind to override what my body was trying to tell me, refusing to take sufficient rest, saying yes to more than I could really cope with, allowing myself to be far more aware of others' needs of me professionally than of my own health and the care I need to be properly available for loved ones.

Wherever you are currently "sitting" in relation to your own ex- periences of anxiety—and how to come into a more appreciative, less hectic way of living—it's all too easy to see why so-called wellness industries are booming. Yet our individual and collective mental health is not. Upping your meditation hours, booking in for more massages, finding someone kind to mind the children for a day, or to fill in for you at your workplace: all of this falls into the category of "nice" (better-than-nothing "nice") that will make little or no difference when the individual experience is over.

> **Anxiety is a state of inner agitation that's a physical crisis as much as a psychological one. It also agitates your experience of the world around you.**

Constant stress, exhaustion, a feeling that you are running without making progress: none of this is sustainable. And the fact that those experiences are shared by millions of others does little to help you. Your situation may be made worse by poor health, financial worries, sexism, racism, feelings of isolation: all disempowering in the here and now.

One of the most effective measures I know is to *ask yourself where your own self-talk is adding to your stress and distress.* And whether *your sense of priorities is thrown into chaos by anxiety or exhaustion.* This is not to blame yourself for the way you feel. On the contrary. But it's where you have the most power to make change.

> *No one but you can make those tough decisions about what matters most.* **What I can say is that the extent to which you can effectively take care of other people, and be with them lovingly and willingly, will be totally dictated by how well you can take care of yourself.**

This doesn't mean ceaseless "me days" (whatever they are). It means not taking on more than you can manage. It means knowing what your values are, and reordering your priorities so that what most directly affects your interdependent circles of people (at home or at work) comes to the top of the list.

It also means *radically adjusting how you feel about doing things*. For example, if you feel like a choiceless martyr, then almost any routine task will seem too much. *Exhaustion adds to this pain*. Prioritizing good food and sleeping soundly, and making time for pleasure and company, are reliable remedies. No time? No opportunity? Self-care and survival say *there must be*.

TRY THIS

Experiment with bringing a different inner narrative to what you do on a daily basis. *This means seeing it as a choice and not as an obligation*.

I'm not suggesting a different attitude when there is even a hint of coercion from another adult. That will *always* require urgent professional attention. This is about *you*—freeing you to be more available to yourself, in addition to any loved ones.

In daily life, there are many things that have to be done. What can change is recognizing that you are not a machine. You are a conscious being, and if you can bring even a tiny amount of conscious awareness and choice to what you are doing, *it will make an enormous difference to your motivation and actions*. No one can make choices for you, or even advise you to "own" your choices, as I seem to be doing. All I can say is that through decades of experience I have seen the power of making such a switch. It is like lighting a little candle in the dark. That tiny light can change everything.

TRY THIS

Let yourself know what causes you excessive stress or anxiety.

- Unpick what "everything" means to you.

- Check how much sleep you are getting: exhaustion makes everything far worse.

- Are you driving yourself hard to impress someone?

- Are you driving yourself hard to silence the Inner Critic?

- Are you self-medicating in ways that can harm you?

- Don't berate yourself. Ever. Speak to yourself like a true friend. Ask yourself, "What small changes would make a difference? How will I make that happen? Do I need help? What's stopping me?"

- Accept offers of help, however imperfect.

- Take mini-breaks throughout each day: taste the water or warm drink you have made. Bring your attention to your breath, and slowly around your body. Can some tension be let go? Would music make a difference? Would a five-minute "nap" slow your thoughts? Would a short walk help, even in the wind or rain?

- You are complex, interesting, unpredictable, and worthy of self-acceptance and encouragement. I strongly suggest these words to loosen your identifications with anxiety and perfectionism. And to help you remind yourself of the truth: "*I unconditionally accept my whole self. I do this with kindness and love.*" Even if you don't "feel like it," these words send a powerful message to your mind, brain, whole self. How could they not?

38 | Self-soothing, self-medicating may make things worse

Congratulations for having the courage to turn to this page. I will write only a part of it. Grabbing that courage, I hope you will write the rest.

The millions of us who feel anxious, overwhelmed, more-than-worried, subject to obsessional catastrophizing and ruminations (whew, quite a list), are likely also to have some favorite habitual distractions. Some of these are better than harmless. Some are exhilarating, delightful, glorious. Some . . . are not.

I'm not referring here to heavy use of alcohol or recreational drugs, gambling, reckless sex, binge-eating, cutting, or other forms of self-harming. You would be wise to seek expert help for any of these. Help is also available from any of the twelve-step programs that work so soundly to loosen the shackles of addiction.

What I have in mind right now is more those overnight television show binges when you are already exhausted, that extra-large block (or two) of chocolate when you aren't hungry, the late-night shopping for clothes you can't really afford.

Or maybe it's unhealthy levels of exercise that strain your heart and wreck your joints? Or resistance to moving off your couch at all? It could be the long, meandering, one-sided conversations with the most patient of your friends. Or the unnecessary criticism of people you envy or dislike. It's often just a "glass or two" (or three or four) too many. Or the well-intended plans made and remade for self-improvement but never translated into action.

Little harm in most of these, but they may be holding you back with limited benefit and—sometimes—creating considerable guilt or intensifying sluggishness or pessimism.

Distracting yourself from anxiety or pain in these ways cannot and will not help you to accept how anxious you are, and *to do something effective about it.*

As with OCD, my strongest plea is that you look for a pattern or patterns in your own behavior, rather than focusing too intensely on a single incident. Look *through the eyes of compassion*, not with harsh or demeaning judgment. Don't punish yourself. Don't guilt-trip yourself. Don't compare your struggles with the hero around the corner or on the screen of your imagination.

> **Read your life thoughtfully. Take back your power as "author." Choose what you will emphasize. Or what you can delegate to a more minor place in your life.**

Ask, "What am I not seeing? What deeper need am I not hearing or heeding? Have I cut myself off from other people? Am I lonely? Am I 'letting in' self-harming or disrespectful or despairing thoughts? What pleasures am I missing? Or bigger engagement with life? Am I tasting the food that's on my plate? Am I walking barefoot sometimes, notic-ing the air on my skin, and where my body is working well—despite 'everything'? Could I breathe a little more slowly and consciously—right now? Could I sit down for my next cup of tea or coffee—and enjoy its flavor and its familiarity? Could I possibly make a plan for something 'out of the ordinary'?"

When you ask yourself such questions, you are tuning in to your inner knowing, your inner wisdom that is so vital to your whole-self perspective. (Writing down your questions, giving yourself heaps of time and permission to "receive" some insights, is always helpful.)

What matters here is re-establishing choice.

Any kind of addictive behavior can be as hard to control in the first instance as fear. Pausing, not acting on impulse, is itself a power-ful means of putting you back in the choice seat. So, when the urge returns to do something that leads you down a familiar path, it's worth a focused moment of self-inquiry: *"What am I feeling right now? What would I prefer to be feeling? What's stopping me?"*

39 | Hannah's story of anxiety and sobriety

This account has been contributed by Hannah M., a writer who lives in Sydney, Australia. These are her words.

There weren't many words to describe mental states or behaviors when I was a child in the 1960s in our deeply religious, slightly paranoid Irish Catholic New Zealand community. "Good" and "naughty" were the primary descriptors of children and their behaviors. Women might have "nervous breakdowns," usually spoken about in a very low voice. Men apparently had no mental issues or any emotional weather to navigate.

Our mother, the adult child of an alcoholic father, was highly anxious, although that word was never used. She feared for the safety of her six children, feared fire in our wooden house, wouldn't let us go into the sea above our knees, feared her own death and our abandonment. ("He will marry again, and no woman can love another woman's children like the mother does.") Despite our father being a sober man, responsible and regular in his attendance at work, due to her childhood experiences she feared financial failure, eviction, poverty, and the police.

She was a woman who dealt with her anxieties not just through what I considered incessant talking but also through prayer—she was a lover of the rosary—and, probably wisely, never sought help from the medical profession for her distress. One of our aunts had suffered a breakdown, and medication rendered her a silent, shuffling zombie. "The cure," our mother remarked, "was worse than the disease."

Poor Mom. I think now how little comfort she had in her life. How brave she was every day. But I only saw the anxiety, not the courage. I continued to resent and resist her control, and her fears. My own anxieties were not apparent to me as I struggled to free myself from hers. If I thought at all about why I started drinking, it was to escape control, to escape limits, to dwell in an expanded space.

I was always looking for transcendence, for the big life. It could not be found (obviously!) in regional New Zealand at the time, and the European dream was still very strong in those days. So, at nineteen, I headed to England, and then at twenty crossed the sea to Ireland where Dublin's pubs opened for me like the celestial gates.

There appeared to be absolutely no controls, no criticisms, and no fears of alcohol. All was warm, cheerful, welcoming: smoky rooms full of desire, music, and endless delightful conversation. And the pubs were so beautiful, with their stained-glass windows and polished wood, and the barman like the priest.

I'd be still there today if it could have stayed like that. If *I* could have stayed like that. I didn't see how I kept being thrown back up and out. It's hard to see the damage being wreaked upon your own body and mind when all you want is the eternal return to the sacred Church/pub.

Months and years went by, and I continued my determined drinking, my drive and dive for depth and grandeur. Within five years I had quit my honest

Dublin job, was on the dole and a meager rent allowance, sucking on roll-your-owns, still ambitious for the big free life while resenting the boyfriend who paid the rent. I was still active in women's causes and trying to write. But anxiety began to stalk me. And depression.

People gave me bits and pieces of work that I could do at home. I was heading for thirty and had nothing to show for it. It was still everyone else's fault. Capitalism. Catholicism. British imperialism. The patriarchy. Mom. The nuns.

Eventually I left Ireland, a land of diminishing returns, and came to Australia to join family members. I celebrated turning thirty in a new country and believed that could pass as progress, as positive change. (A return to New Zealand felt impossible—a sign of true defeat.) And anyway I believed that no one there could cope with a broken person. Psychic pain would be ignored, and a torrent of trivial story would just flow over me.

I put down alcohol in Sydney. Under the great blue skies, I started to breathe a little easier. In a way I had to give up drinking as even one glass of champagne led to an instant mood swing (down!) and diarrhea. I found tai chi, plus paid work that nearly drove me mad with boredom. I decided to go to university.

Not drinking certainly meant an improvement in what could be done in life, but I still had lots of fears. Fears of the future were huge. As in childhood, I had a feeling I couldn't do "ordinary life" and kept hoping for some form of special exemption pass.

I started a degree as a mature-age student and loved it. I loved the vastness of an arts degree and I made friends. Some of us started a writers' group and journal. Life was rich although I was poor, but I feared life after college. What would I do? Where would I go? How could I do interviews? How would I know what was required? One day in a history professor's office I had an eerie sensation that I was standing on very thin ice. I looked down and saw solid floor beneath me, which slightly eased the sense of panic, but I understood the message.

On a scale of 0 to 10, my levels of anxiety at that time were around 7 or 8. But I thought that was normal. I began smoking again, and that sort of helped. It was one of my new university friends who "twelve-stepped" me into the program, not into AA [Alcoholics Anonymous] but into Al-Anon, because as he said, "You don't drink yet you exhibit all the signs of alcoholism." Which, he went on to inform me, were solitude in the midst of the crowd, apparently super sociability but a refusal of intimacy, driven to achieve, and high anxiety.

After one year of Al-Anon I went to my first AA meeting and found the physical sense of something within me truly easing as I walked into my first of AA's many shabby halls and gentle circles, with their interplay of humor and grief. A very deep sense of relief within persisted after the meeting, which was why I returned and still keep returning. I had finally gotten somewhere safe and true. Who knows, I might even begin to relax and let go of the expectation to be superhuman, the desire to not feel anything except the highs and satisfactions of life, the fear of failure, the perfectionism: all the hallmarks of the emotionally immature alcoholic; all leading to anxiety.

It's the third step of AA that provides me with the most help with my anxiety: "Made a decision to turn our will and our lives over to the care of God *as we understand God.*" The italicized emphasis in that step is AA's—not mine. It is one of AA's most liberating tenets: Go ahead and choose your own conception of God. Then there's the acronym TRUST: "Try Really Using Step Three," proposed by some member. Once I might have resisted the folksy collective wisdoms of the program. Now I know I don't have to resist. I am free to choose.

The Sufis say, "Abjure the why, and seek the how." All alcoholics have an origin story and are encouraged by the program to construct, understand, and retell their own narrative. This may include genetics, childhood, or other trauma. But the emphasis is on *how do we heal these broken selves?* How do we hope to live in this perplexing world of (apparent) adults when we feel like children? How do we get on with today? The answer—and the emphasis, of course—is on "just for today." *"It is only when you and I add the burden of those two awful eternities, yesterday and tomorrow, that we break down."* The answer is also *acceptance*.

In the company of AA, with its community networks, its friendships, its written and spoken guidance, its variety of meetings, its encouragement, understanding, and the way you get to speak at meetings *without interruption*, (and people are asked to not give you feedback or advice—hallelujah!), I have progressed in my journey through the so-called real world.

Eventually I gave up smoking. I could not have done that without AA. Once I let go of nicotine, I realized how much it had been "holding the fort" of my alcoholism. The experience of giving up cigarettes was dramatic—an excruciating and a life-enhancing process—colors, sounds, insights all seemed to be at an increased internal volume. And the beauty of the world!

Recovery for me has been an increasing awareness of that beauty. As well as improving my stamina in the work of creating things. And learning to trust the hunches, the intuitions, and the job offers. Learning to say "Yes" to life. I've joined choirs, learned how to garden and knit, written four books in recovery, completed a PhD, repaired relationships with siblings and my dear parents, been in love twice, bought a flat, and been kept busy and happy in paid work that utilizes my writing and communicative powers. I've been present for the dying processes of both my parents and tried to be present for the challenges that my siblings and friends face.

There have been times when my anxiety has broken through. Once, traveling overseas on my own, I had overestimated my personal emotional resources and was finding it very difficult to continue. Beauty was all around me but I couldn't feel it. I felt slowed, almost paralyzed by anxiety.

A group member made the comment in a soothing email that my anxiety was trying to be helpful. It had given itself, "The noble task of keeping you safe." That was a liberating insight for me. My anxiety was not my enemy, just a fearful but possibly even sweet and caring—if very annoying—friend.

Sobriety can protect you from the wounded subconscious which alcohol lays you wide open to, but it is not meant to cover it up. I still have outbreaks of anxiety, depression, obsessional thinking. The point is, in AA we continue to do our daily stuff. And attend meetings. Or talk to people. Or read spiritual literature. And pray or meditate. Do the practices. We say, "Having a shit time. Haunted at the moment. Boxed in. *Sad.* Bitten by the past." Whose past is not always clear. Weep if we can. Write if we can't. Writing gets to it. Writing helps heal "it," for me.

I'm very grateful to be in a twelve-step community that can laugh as we support one another to keep breathing and keep walking through this life, facing things, but *not like a superhero.* Like a human allowed to go to bed when she's overwhelmed, encouraged to call a friend—or acquaintance—to share the story of fear or indecision or rage or obsessional rat-in-a-trap thinking. Or call on the Higher Power, the Universe, the Mystery, the Great Mother: whoever and whatever. Call on the dead or the living or the utterly transformed. Just call.

I deal with my alcoholic anxieties in sobriety today with honesty and comfort. Truth in my daily life frees me from many fears, including the fear of speaking the truth. But I also need to comfort the fearful one within. Physical comforts include warm baths, clean sheets, massages, foot soaks, (anything that hugs, strokes, soothes), cups of tea, garden sits. Twelve-step literature helps, AA's, Al-Anon's, Melody Beattie, as well as soothing spiritual writing such as poetry. I find in times of anxiety the call to spiritual heroism found in some self-help or esoteric texts does *not* work.

Prayer helps. (Who'd have thought!) My wooden Sufi prayer beads have done the rounds many times in the middle of the night, and yes, praying for others is very soothing. Each bead is a prayer for a friend, colleague, a neighbor, a family member, or the people in the local shops. By the time I get to the end of the beads, I am cheered by the thought of all the good people in the world. If the mind is still not settled, I do another round. *And I pray for myself.* I am allowed to care for and comfort myself. That old stern religion is gone. There's a new one of love, beauty, creativity, service to others. And kindness to all.

40 | From childhood to adolescence

If you are involved with children and young people, there may be no greater gift to share than trust in themselves as a whole person or self. It's this that will support them to hold on to a more generous picture of themselves even when things go wrong, as they inevitably will. It is also the basis of genuine resilience: "I can and will cope." A self-respecting attitude will let them take pleasure in their efforts—without feeling their self-confidence is wholly dependent on flying higher than anyone around them.

A whole-self experience that embraces all of who you are is necessary to counteract the binary thinking that harms us socially and personally. This is the thinking that can divide the world into "us" and "them," that can split us off from ourselves, allowing us to obsess about "what's wrong" while overlooking strengths that are just as much a part of us.

On small and big issues, reductive thinking causes havoc to our internal integrity and social cohesion. Anxiety is a response to this misery.

Our own eyes as well as global data show us anxiety among children and adolescents is increasing, including in serious forms like OCD, self-harm, risk-taking behaviors around sex or drugs or alcohol, or suicide or suicidal ideation. As Linda's story about Mark's OCD shows (in chapter 42), adequate treatment is difficult to find and out of reach for too many families.

Linda's story shows something else, too. Even in a conventionally stable household, children can suffer disabling anxiety in its many forms. How could they not? They, too, live in an anxious, ruthless, often violent world. They, too, are subject to the stresses of competitiveness, social anxiety, and wider social injustice. They, too, may have genetic or temperamental factors playing a part. Yet lazy assumptions continue to be made about what the "perfect household" looks like. Or the "perfect circumstances" to avoid mental illness or trauma.

> **Anxiety in any child's life can be overwhelming, especially when it expresses as intense fear of separation, change, or panic around circumstances that can't be fully predicted. "I just need to know what's happening" makes perfect sense to the weeping child—and any older person, too.**

It makes sense, too, that while many anxious children may be shy or socially withdrawn, others will be irritable, subject to angry outbursts that may shame them, and certainly to depression along with anxiety.

It seems *all* children and many adults would benefit from routines and predictable rhythms that need not be set in stone to be comforting but do bring the boundaries necessary to feel safe. Those boundaries may well be around screen time, or what is watched. They may involve bedtimes, mealtimes, meeting deadlines without panic, and adults making decisions with calm good humor. For many children that is essential.

Children are subject to their own stresses and are also highly vulnerable to the stresses of their parents or carers, *which they cannot influence or control.*

Slowing down the pace of the household, enjoying nature in parks, gardens, beaches—jumping in the rain—making time for anything that is creative or expressive, making time for lots of chatting even when the dishes aren't done and the washing isn't folded—those shifts in priority are felt by children. And they benefit instantly from them. It doesn't have to mean no time on screens, but no screen delivers life firsthand.

As I routinely emphasize, play down rote learning, anxious competitiveness, the importance of the next "test." This is pedagogy at its worst. Encourage fascination, wonder, awe, experiential learning of every kind. Encourage friendships, and eating together—and talking while eating. Put food out on large plates in the center, however simple, so that children learn to help others to it, as well as to chat while they help themselves. Shop, cook, plan meals together. Be adventurous there, too. Expand "likes."

Understanding what causes most stress in your household is basic. Perhaps the demands of the school are unreasonable. Or your child isn't feeling accepted or included by others. And where there is poverty, racism, or a breakdown of warmth between the parents or carers, professional help is essential.

**Stress creates anxiety and worsens it, *whatever your age.*
Stress tells you that everything is an emergency—
and there's no time to be happy.**

**Stress tells you that if something is not totally
perfect, then it is totally wrong.
Stress robs you of this moment (that will never come again),
pushing you ruthlessly toward the next and the next.**

Young people who are questioning their sexuality or gender, or who belong to a minority community stereotyped in the media, will be at increased risk of anxiety, depression, and self-harm. The emotional shelter and acceptance their parents or carers can provide is crucial in a world where ignorance still prevails.

It is a national shame that First Nations young people in Australia are at a significantly higher risk of mental illness and suicide than non-Indigenous people. After the age of fifteen, nearly one-third of First Nations people are at high to very high risk of psychological distress. This is echoed in all ex-colonies, like Canada and New Zealand, and inescapably demonstrates that social disadvantage and structural discrimination have profound effects down through the generations. A very similar picture exists in the United States among Native Americans, while Black or African American people of all ages name racism among the top three concerns affecting their mental health. *How could this be otherwise?*

Nothing is more important than speaking up about the structural disadvantages that affect millions of children, most particularly race but also education and health systems that fail too many, the widespread acceptance of violence as entertainment, as well as housing and food insecurity: unforgivable betrayals of children.

For children in wealthier circumstances, the pressures of status and body anxiety, social media exposure, competitiveness, pressures to perform and conform can also preoccupy young minds and make it more difficult to *trust their intrinsic worth*. (I feel very, very strongly about constant "testing" in any school setting. This happens in some public and private schools with children as young as five. It elevates rote learning above gaining knowledge. It fails the basic test of emotional intelligence, which is learning to cooperate, not compete, with others. Children are not lab rats!)

My bias is always toward developing the lifelong values of cooperation, curiosity, love of nature, interest in other people, team sports, and creative arts, including daily music, that are sociable, exuberant, inclusive. Am I talking about having fun? Yes! As Bill Bryson writes in *A Walk in the Woods*, "All over America today people would be dragging themselves to work, stuck in traffic jams, wreathed in exhaust smoke. I was going for a walk in the woods."

Life is not a continuous "walk in the woods," and we might appreciate it less if it were. We will face challenges, *whoever we are*. So will the children and adolescents we love. Adults can encourage resilience, especially by the way they talk about their own challenges—and *how they talk about themselves*.

Habits of putting yourself down ("I'm an idiot . . ."), criticizing your physical self ("I hate my body . . ."), being routinely critical of other people ("I work with a bunch of losers . . ."), predicting doom ("Try if you want to, but I wouldn't . . ."), or "drowning sorrows" in the bottom of a glass will always be observed by any children or young people around you. The greatest support we can give to others is showing (not telling) our eagerness to live fully and appreciatively. And doing that.

41 | Elena's story (aged fifteen)

Anxiety is something so many of us struggle with.

ELENA

Elena is a high-school student living in an expensive, hectic, major city. Her account offers a great deal of insight into what anxiety—and life— feels like for a young woman her age living as she does at a time of significant change and uncertainty. As she herself says, each person's experiences are unique, yet telling our stories has always been an essential way to support others and to feel less alone. Listening and talking across the generations is essential for our well-being, perhaps our survival.

Elena says that some of the feelings of anxiety from her childhood have been replaced by feelings maybe more akin to depression, though she adds, "That sounds pretty dramatic. Possibly just moody instead. Still, the feeling of frequent not-belonging has persisted, and while it has never been a cause of anxiety, it has been a cause of loneliness, maybe in turn causing other spurts of depression/anxiety."

She also explained in a separate conversation that anxiety is probably experienced differently by "people who are more focused on grades, or appearance, or relationships, or popularity, and maybe less focused on the broader future, internal pursuits, their own groups of friends and people they hold close." Elena's story continues in her words.

I don't think of myself as a generally anxious person. I am usually able to stay quite calm about most things and try not to make possibly stressful situations into mental catastrophes. However, yes, there are some situations that I find are more worrying than others, most of them related to things like school and interactions with other people my age. I think it is a mix of how I am perceived as well as how I am doing things, and they bounce off each other a bit. Like, for example, I'm going to a class at school I don't really have any friends in, I either sit alone or awkwardly near some other group, and am perceived as being friendless or an intruder, and then become hyperaware of what I am doing.

When I overthink and become hyper-aware, I do things differently from how I normally would, spending more time *thinking* about how someone would act casually in this situation rather than just acting casually. The two (being perceived wrongly/oddly and acting differently) make this awful sort of mixing pot, and just kind of spiral together.

Then there are things like the broader future, climate change, whether I will ever be able to move out of home in this city (a premature worry and a little sarcastic, but you get the idea), and other "big" concerns.

My anxiety levels have definitely changed since I was a young child. I used to be extremely anxious about basically everything, a phase I have since outgrown. I'm not sure if there is a single most striking change, since almost everything has changed drastically, but I've learned as I get older and move schools and meet new friends to just take it as it goes and try not to meticulously plan everything out. Especially for things I have no control over, and that planning out and worrying over would do nothing for.

Weirdly enough, moving schools several times has helped me. I've moved around a little bit, seen lots of friends come and go, and have started to understand that for better or worse things always change. Getting too fixed on making sure everything is right "right now" is kind of futile because, like I said earlier, a lot of it is out of my control.

The areas of my life most intruded upon by anxiety usually involve the broader future. The years ahead I am not yet able to imagine or comprehend. I know I've spoken a bit about how I try not to stress over things coming and going so much, but when it comes to my adult years, so far ahead, it's pretty different. The climate crisis, for example, with a lot of my generation leaning to the more cynical side and being fully convinced that we don't really have a future, with rising temperatures and sea levels and deforestation, and the immense feeling of helplessness even though it is something that will very deeply affect my life, is a cause of great anxiety.

I'm probably least intruded upon by anxiety by current friend groups and teachers and grades and other adolescent things that I do certainly care about—I can't think of many aspects of my life that I *don't* care about—but that I don't let the fate of these friendships and classes and things give me cause for real concern, especially when I could be doing other things, and nothing seems presently wrong.

It's not always easy to encourage myself. I tend to clam up and just cave in on myself a bit before remembering that this will end, change, shift, whatever, and just wait it out and remember that I have friends and family I can talk to if needs be. Often, I don't though. I feel very strongly about something in one moment, but by the time I'm able to text or talk to someone about it, the feeling is subdued, and I don't feel like talking.

As for other people confiding in me, I think the older I get the easier I am to talk to, but actually getting to know me, no, I don't think that's easy. Only some people really do, and those people are generally just the ones I'm close to and the people I like the most. I'm glad I'm getting better at simply talking to people, but I don't necessarily want to show off different parts of me to just anyone. However, I do wish that when I get to the point that I *think* someone knows me very well, that they managed to prove it and didn't let me down as much.

My best ways to relax are talking to and seeing the people I'm close with, writing, reading, listening to music, recovering by lounging around the house and watching my favorite shows, just generally things I enjoy. I can be open with my family and my close friends. I'm pretty lucky about that, and I know it's not that way for everyone my age.

I know I keep repeating myself, but I get hope from the knowledge that things will change, this will be different, that the people who I want to stick with and who want to stick with me I can continue to stay close with (I know this after moving schools a bit). But mostly I get hope from the fact that my situation as a teenager is a temporary one that doesn't define my life or future or anything.

Almost everyone I know my age—or the girls at least—are advocates for being open about your mental health, especially with anxiety, something so many of us struggle with. I see some people, some girls at school, that seem to be able to click with other people so easily and manage to like the same things as everybody else, and think the same things as everybody else, and have a good time while doing it. Which is not to say they're not individuals, or that they're not as "cool" or "smart" as I am, just that they really do seem to like what other people like and behave the same way. So, it's as if they never have to worry about not feeling like they belong, or being isolated, which makes school and adolescence look incredibly simple for them.

Still, I know from knowing some of these girls that this is not always the case, and the same inner turmoil seems to exist within most of us, no matter what clothes you wear or what music and shows and makeup you like or don't like, or how many friends you have.

I do really understand that a single instance or trait does not define us, nor does a moment, an emotion or feeling we are susceptible to have to become all of us. That being said, anxiety can have a huge influence on how a person acts, I know from experience, so it can almost seem as if anxiety is what a person has become, simply because of how much it's tainted anything else. Same goes for other mental health issues.

Things like writing help me cope, whether it's good or bad, just to get something on a page, which definitely helps to subdue whatever pain I'm feeling, as well as actually talking to others about my problems when I need to. I've always been lucky enough to have people I can turn to when I have to, and have always felt comfortable enough to do so, given the supportive family in which I have been raised. And writing is something that I feel has come naturally, whether it takes the form of a short story or even just a diary entry, spilling my guts onto a page has always made me feel better.

A further change? Maybe opening myself up more. Maybe getting better in social situations at not closing in on myself sometimes? I do, however, feel that these are things I've improved on in myself over the years, without help from therapy. *Writing works for me.*

42 | A parent's story of OCD

When someone is severely affected by anxiety, it will shape most or all aspects of their life. It will also affect their closest people, family, and friends. In those toughest times, compassionate and informed support is needed. Yet the reality is that professional support can be hard to access and may be patchy at best. And many families, friends, siblings, and partners feel ill-equipped to judge what the "right thing to do" may be.

The "right thing"—in my experience—is usually to remain as open-minded as possible, as well as open-hearted. Dogmatic opinions close us off to other possibilities. It is also useful for sufferers and for carers to examine their assumptions about anxiety: they may be way off the mark. We are all individuals. *Nothing is more unique than a person's psyche.* We are certainly not a statistic. Your experience or mine may not be represented in any data.

Continuing to respect the individuality of a loved one is vital. Continuing (stubbornly) to trust an innate leaning within ourselves toward healing is sustaining. I need to note, too, that mental health services in most countries are woefully inadequate, most particularly for minorities, for children and adolescents, and especially for those without access to private insurance and the time and money to pursue a variety of options. Structural inequalities, racism, and sexism *cause anxiety as well as worsen it*. Yet, as the following story shows, the most considerate and stable family cannot wholly protect their loved ones. Or themselves.

The mother who tells the story below has been generously frank in order to support others reading her account in this book. She lives in New England in the United States, but has wisely chosen to be discreet about further identifying details, for the sake of her whole family, and particularly for the son who suffered from OCD. Here I am calling her Linda, and her son Mark. These are Linda's words.

In hindsight, we did not notice any anxiety much in Mark until about age three. Infant and toddler behaviors were very typical of "normal," non-anxious children that age. There'd been no significant anxiety for either his dad or me. I had one window as I approached thirty when I had some panic attacks that were well controlled and addressed in therapy. But I consider any anxiety that we faced as pretty typical of most people.

I don't think our son's OCD came out of the blue. I think there was a process throughout his preschool and younger elementary years when certain stressors were apparent. He was a bit of an outlier on and off in school social settings, although he always very much wanted to be a part of it all. I'm not sure if the younger children picked up on some of his anxiety, which they may have seen as strange. Maybe this contributed to him not being fully embraced in social settings outside of our friend/family group where he was loved.

In fifth grade Mark faced significant bullying and I definitely think that time frame played a role in pushing him over the edge into more symptomatic OCD. We ended up moving him to a different school for sixth grade and it was that year when certain (contamination) triggers got instilled into his thought patterns. This ultimately led to significant OCD symptoms in the fall of seventh grade when he was twelve years old.

That year, his OCD became very intrusive and life-altering fairly quickly. In fifth grade, there had been incidents of excessive handwashing that resulted in dry, chapped hands. However, as we live in New England, that can be a common occurrence in our dry, cold weather. Again, that is one of the red flags we picked up on in hindsight.

Our son's OCD revolved around contamination issues. He was showering for several hours a day and was very agitated when he wasn't cleaning himself. The compulsions greatly interfered with his ability to attend school or to go to bed at night. We were extremely concerned by this point.

I have a master's degree in social work that provided me with minimal training about OCD. I did recognize our son's symptoms and diagnosed his OCD myself. I sought a therapist in our area who claimed to specialize in the treatment of OCD. She was not qualified at all, and now that I know so much about OCD and its treatment, I realize the couple of months working with her were a waste of time. After several sessions with her I realized she was not helpful for us. She discouraged my pursuit of outside professional resources repeatedly and thought small assignments like using five pumps of soap instead of seven when washing yourself would work if given time. Instead, our son grew increasingly consumed with his compulsions.

That was a frustrating time because very few people seemed to understand or know how to properly treat severe OCD. We consulted with a psychiatrist at our area hospital who started Mark on a low dose of Prozac. This ended up not being the correct medication or dosage to manage his symptoms. Luckily, we had a wonderful pediatrician who put her ego aside and acknowledged that she had limited resources to help us. She encouraged my efforts to find help for our son.

I used my experience in social work to seek out other resources in the United States. At that time, there were only two inpatient treatment centers for children that could treat the significant level of OCD our son was suffering. They were McLean Hospital in Boston and Rogers Behavioral Health in Wisconsin.

McLean had a very lengthy wait. As we witnessed Mark in significant crisis, we knew he would get worse and worse without an aggressive intervention. Luckily, Rogers alerted us fairly quickly that they could take him in early December because many opted out of entering the program during the holiday season. I did extensive intake work with them on the phone prior to our arrival. Our son's score on the Yale-Brown OCD scale was 36/40, which is their highest ranking. His compulsions were still around contamination and there were very few times in the day when his obsessive thoughts and the resulting compulsions were not intruding. These thoughts are essentially delusional, insisting to the sufferer that nothing matters more than fulfilling compulsive demands. There was little or no respite for Mark during this time.

I had originally hoped he could do daily outpatient work but was informed that he would need to be an inpatient. That was a horribly sad and challenging time because we hated the idea of having to leave him at a residential treatment center for a month or longer. The next emotional blow was when they informed us that his treatment length would be closer to eighty days. We did not share details with Mark at first because he was so overwhelmed by his OCD. He knew we were moving temporarily to Wisconsin so that he would get help. Once we arrived there, we had to inform him of the residential component of his treatment.

He was initially very frightened and worried that we would return to New England without him. As the weeks progressed and he was finally getting the help he needed, his fears about our leaving and his unhappiness to sleep there without us decreased. He ended up making some nice friends who also lived there with him, and they provided another layer of support to one another.

We rented a house next to the hospital. Mark was twelve, and our younger son, aged seven, also relocated with us. I homeschooled our younger son during his brother's treatment. Our moving cross-country to get treatment was unusual, but we felt strongly that we would tackle this illness together, supporting one another each step of the way. I know this helped Mark feel stronger to fight back against his OCD. It also allowed us, as the ones closest to him, to deep dive into everything OCD and be better prepared going forward to understand the disorder and its treatment.

He was the only child in the facility who had parents that relocated to be nearby full-time. I understand what we did is not possible for most families. We were fortunate that I was not working outside the home and my husband had a job that he was able to do via his computer from our rental.

Being nearby allowed us to participate on a daily basis in our son's treatment with his extremely qualified treatment team. While unusual to have families be a part of daily therapy, the staff embraced our active roles each day. The main focus of treatment for OCD at Rogers was exposure response prevention (ERP) therapy. ERP therapy was tough. It forced Mark to do various things that made him feel contaminated and sit with the tremendous anxiety that ensued. He had to do this consistently throughout the day with his therapist, his caretakers at the dormitory, and with us. It did get a little easier for him as time passed.

Mark also had medical doctors at Rogers who prescribed him an SSRI [selective serotonin reuptake inhibitor, or antidepressant]. His dose was gradually increased while he was there. When we transitioned back home, medication continued to play a huge role in his treatment. It was not until several years later that we finally found his sweet spot for both dosage and brand. For Mark, a daily SSRI has proven to be an ongoing essential piece of his OCD management.

While we were in Wisconsin, all of us did individual therapy as well as family therapy. Our son had daily individual and group therapy with the other kids in his treatment program as well. Rogers held weekly parent seminars to educate and support the parents of their inpatient residents. For these meetings, other parents would drive or fly in for a one- or two-day visit. Spending time in individual therapy and group therapy gave each of us insights into our own trauma that resulted from Mark's OCD, as well as many tools to help Mark going forward. This was another resource that we were fortunate to be able to access that might not be as accessible to others. Our flexible schedules during that time were certainly unusual and not realistic for many.

While many couples fall apart with the immeasurable stress having a sick child brings into a marriage, the experience strengthened our relationship. We were truly a team. When one of us needed to tag out, the other stepped in. It became apparent we each brought unique and critical strengths to our partnership. I am the researcher showrunner, while my husband is calm and steady. Without each other I'm not sure how well either of us would have handled it. Inevitably, it changed our family and our parenting style. We have a very tight nuclear family at least in part because of what we have been through together. Similarly, we all know that each of us is 100 percent there for each other. I also think it's given the four of us a strength going forward because we got through this truly awful low period together.

Watching a sick older brother go through such a painful and scary time did impact my younger son. He is flourishing now, though, so it did not cause significant, long-term harm. There was a time when I think he worried he might get sick, but he had therapy, and we as a family have always spoken very openly so his concerns did pass. I believe that time has been the most important factor. It has been half a lifetime ago for our younger son, so it is not a part of his thoughts anymore.

Ironically there are some good things that came from all the pain. Mark, nine years after our stay at Rogers, is very resilient. The four years following his inpatient treatment were still filled with lots of work around his OCD and lots of ups and downs in school and socially. He has seen and experienced some of the worst life throws at you, and he has survived. That has been a powerful lesson for him, and I often witness the impact that survival trait has on obstacles he encounters now.

Both our boys have seen that their parents, grandparents, and close family friends love them and support them unconditionally. That gives them a sense of security and confidence that may or may not have been as evident had we not experienced this period in our lives.

What helped most? Lots of therapy. Lots of professional support and guidance. Rogers helped us transition from their care to our life. We had a wonderful therapist who came to our home regularly as soon as our son was done at Rogers. Through the International OCD Foundation (IOCDF; https://iocdf.org/) we found the only trained ERP psychologist in our region. He was a part of our lives and we saw him regularly for seven years. He recently retired and because our son's OCD has now been in remission for several years, we sadly said goodbye.

Given our son's current remission status, he does not currently want or need regular therapy. We do, though, have a wonderful doctor at a leading medical institute in New York City, as well as access to his colleagues as needed. We see him three times a year, and he manages Mark's continuing medication. Having the proper dosage and type of SSRI has proven invaluable.

Now that we are well past that crisis time, I would say bullying and a somewhat anxious, sensitive predisposition led to the emergence of Mark's OCD. An important lesson I learned from our long-term family therapist is that almost everyone has anxiety, and many people are on the spectrum for OCD. He pointed out that it is only when the anxiety from OCD is interfering with one's quality of life that it is problematic. Who knows if my son's OCD would have become so severe had outside factors been different. Getting to Rogers was the game changer for us and connecting with professionals who knew how to treat OCD. We have had access to experts ever since, so have had help as needed.

Obviously, I now know more about OCD than I ever wanted to know. I think all of us are more compassionate toward people struggling with mental health issues because we've been there. Following that crisis, I was fearful for a long time. Thankfully, our son has been in remission now for several years, and we are thankful to be in a place where none of us needs to think much about OCD. I've been told by many providers over the years that aggressive early treatment has a good prognosis. I also understand and greatly sympathize that this is not always the case. Many do not have access to what we did. And many cases aren't as responsive to treatment. In the big picture, I guess we were some of the lucky ones. But I don't want that to take away from the tremendous amount of work that Mark himself did to aid his recovery. He was very determined, and it was very hard work. He just kept plowing through and he got to the other side.

I know it's possible that issues could arise again. We also know that we would address anything that comes up very promptly, and with highly qualified care. Having a continued close relationship with the team in New York City gives us access to help right away if needed, and having that resource, and knowing OCD as well as we do, has made it less scary. As our son has moved from adolescence to adulthood, he appears no more anxious than most people around his age. He has good friends and now lives and works in New York City totally independently. We remain grateful for the help we could get and eager for this debilitating disorder to be far better understood and treated.

Part Four

Insight and action

43 | Start with the big picture

Keep some room in your heart for the unimaginable.

MARY OLIVER

Long before you consider "what to do" about anxiety, you may need to look with new eyes at the far more basic issue of "who you are." *Who you are.* What makes you a complex, ever-changing, unique individual, such as we all are. You may need to discover how to locate a bigger picture of yourself that is so much more than the view that anxiety brings. And you may need to discover what's possible when you can detach even somewhat from habits of seeing (or talking about) yourself that are in any way limiting.

When anxiety has you in its grip, that grip can be crushing. That's because anxiety in its many forms skews the way you interpret events and experiences. It affects your relationships. It undermines your resilience. It can make you uncomfortably reliant on other people's praise or fickle acceptance. It tells you sneaky lies about your competence. It tells you that you can't afford to fail. Or that your "successes" don't count.

Habits of self-criticism are cruel. So is a paralyzing fear of change, or of how other people see you. You may dread the nights, suffering versions of night terrors, or debilitating sleeplessness. Or it could be that waking up to yet another day is what's hardest.

Any or all of those states of mind come with the territory of "anxious." And much more besides. But, as I continue to repeat, in the mix of our psychological challenges, *anxiety is the most treatable*. What's more, when at least some of this "treating" comes from a regaining of your personal power *through your own insights and changed attitudes*, there's a double victory.

Establishing a more generous attitude to yourself will not "disappear" anxiety or your heightened sensitivities all at once. *What it will do is put anxiety in its place: uncomfortable sometimes, maybe hard to bear occasionally, but never a life sentence.*

When you are used to looking at life through the prism of anxiety, it can be quite startling to seek and find a truer, more encompassing, whole-self "view." You could liken it to looking through the narrowing end of a telescope, then switching to the vast view of what a telescope can actually reveal.

> **This kind of relaxed, nonjudgmental self-awareness**
> **decreases tension in your body.** *It also helps greatly*
> *in re-establishing your mind as an ally, as a friend, when*
> *it has seemed to be a source of persistent distress.*

While "making friends" again with your mind might sound trivial or ridiculous, it can quickly be experienced as a source of quiet inner steadying that you have access to at all times.

TRY THIS

Imagination has brought you some of your worst moments. Now it can support you. Take a few minutes right now to put down your book, close your eyes, and visualize yourself in any situation where you were enthusiastic, unselfconscious, engaged, or inspired. Or just chilling and feeling quietly content.

Take your time. Enjoy those images and memories (even if they seem "long ago" or fleeting). Let them remind you of the bigger, more complex person than anxiety suggests you are. Look for details. Notice how your body feels as you offer yourself acceptance, how you are breathing, how your face looks when you are excited or relaxed, what the sounds are around you, the feel of air on your skin, or the chill of a bracing day.

To enter this scene, let go of some of your assumptions. There's adventurousness and curiosity in that. Your mind is bringing you gifts, even if briefly.

Take in a sense of being "in place," of your *wholeness*: the aspects of yourself you can see; the aspects that you can't see but you sense and feel.

Add words if you feel so inclined: *"Whatever difficulties I face, I wholly and completely accept myself." "I accept myself just as I am." "The door of my heart is open." "I accept my whole self." "I am grateful."*

Return to that inner picture or something similar as often as you need to. It is a gentle prompt to bring positive images to mind. It makes the unimaginable imaginable.

44 | Self-care basics

Caring for myself is not self-indulgence, it is self-preservation.
AUDRE LORDE

Essential to self-care is feeling safe (and real) within your own self, together with a confidence that it is safe for you to be at least somewhat connected to other people and *accepted by them.* There's definitely a sweet spot between being too self-involved—leaning toward babying yourself or even narcissism—and not self-caring enough. Finding that sweet spot matters. Unless you have some acquaintance with treating yourself respectfully and thoughtfully, your stance in the world will feel shaky. So will your relationships with other people.

Self-care depends on attitude. Two insight questions that are basic to self-care can, or should, become central to your daily routines. The first is one to be asked whenever you question how your behaviors or innermost thoughts are affecting you or others. It is, *"Is this kind?"*

The second question is *"What's stopping me?"* That's for when you know change is needed—but . . . somehow old habits are keeping you stuck, pinned like a butterfly: still beautiful but unable to use your wings.

What's also central to self-care is a determination not to be ruled by feelings that may be working against you, and not for you. Does that strike you as strange? Your feelings matter, yes. Yet feelings reflect *emotional* patterns of response. They can easily take you in anything but a caring direction.

Take a hint from Morita therapy: as you act positively—doing what needs to be done—your feelings will change. Don't ask yourself, "Do I feel like it?" when it comes to self-care and self-and-others caring basics. William James was an early psychologist and brother of the famous writer, Henry James. He suggested that "the great thing, then, in all education, is to make our nervous system our ally instead of our enemy." James died in 1910 and could have had no idea how poignantly his words would resound more than a hundred years later. *To make an "ally" of your nervous system—as well as of your mind—is a profound act of self-cherishing, most particularly when we are also learning, slowly, how necessary it is to cherish all of life, and one another.*

Taking charge of what captures your time and attention, *moving forward,* making an ally of all your "systems"—including "nervous"—these are choices with tremendously positive consequences. Your anxious feelings can be acknowledged. You may still need support. But in these daily ways, you will see yourself far less as an "anxious person," far more as a choosing, whole, flourishing self.

Let your self-care "basics" *be* basic, be the foundation, be the steadying you need.

1. Anxiety is treatable, but you will do best by seeing yourself as *the key member of your treating team.*

2. *Make your relationships a top priority.* Your mental health depends on feeling connected.

3. You cannot deal with anxiety effectively without carefully assessing where life is bringing more stress than you can deal with. We live in a cruelly stressful world where people compete about how "tough" they are emotionally. This is madness. *Refuse to play that game.*

4. How can your life have many more moments of delight, discovery? Make this a high priority.

5. Eat as well as you can. Avoid sugar and processed food. Go for natural, delicious tastes. Eat consciously so that you are enjoying it—and your mind is not many miles away from your mouth.

6. Exercise for pleasure, not just fitness.

7. However hard it first seems, speak to and about yourself appreciatively. And *verbalize your appreciation of other people*—daily. Switching from a critical mind to an appreciative one, you change your world.

8. Sleep will always be disturbed when your cortisol levels are too high (or too low, according to Gabor Maté in *The Myth of Normal*). Sleep is also dramatically disturbed when your mind is overwhelmed by worries, internal conflicts, or fears that life is getting worse. Everything in this book points toward easing those burdens. A first step, always, is to put some kind of clear boundary around them. Write in your journal or the notebook by your bed, "Today I have done all that I can. Tomorrow I will . . ." Then list *no more than three actions*, at least one of which *also takes care of you.*

45 | The power of venting

Let's assume you can't bear one more hard or horrible thing happening. Then one more thing does happen. It may be a disappointment. It might be that your symptoms of anxiety or depression are suddenly worse. Or your chronic pain becomes acute. Perhaps you are not going to get the job or promotion you were counting on. It could be that you are wounded by someone's rudeness, their misreading of you, or worse. Someone you love is falling in a heap and you are powerless to help.

If what is happening internally is significantly worsening your physical or emotional health, do not wait. Get the medical help you need as quickly as you can. This may mean going to a trusted family doctor. It may also mean calling on emergency mental health crisis services. Use the "heart attack" rule as your measure. If you know someone has heart problems that seem significantly worse, would you hesitate to call for help—even if it means "inconveniencing" others, or risking that things will settle "in their own time"?

I would also strongly suggest that your "safety net" preparations for a crisis include *medical advice in advance*. You are *not* more likely to "make something happen" by being sensibly prepared for it. You are less likely, knowing that you are not alone—and even if "help" is not perfect, you do know how to go about accessing it.

If what is happening in your own mind and emotions is more about others' behavior that feels unjust, unfair, crushing, it will quickly become overwhelming if *you are already feeling vulnerable.*

When a situation feels "too much," it probably is. *We all have limits to our resilience.* Anyone who believes they can cope with whatever comes hasn't yet experienced an emotional tsunami. Maybe not much of a ripple, either.

So, what can help you when one more thing arrives, confirming your foreboding that *everything* goes wrong? And *nothing* ever goes right?

It may not be popular, but I would say most of us will need to vent. Initially. Strongly. Unreasonably. (You may also need to run, take a brief, very cold shower, or throw yourself into some other fairly exhausting, distracting physical activity. Venting, though, is also a tension release, a "steam" release—taking pressure from you and "putting it out there.")

What venting means is pouring out all those sad, angry, disappointed, let-down feelings without feeling guilty that there are indeed billions worse off, and you have no right to complain. The ideal person to vent with is your therapist. They are being paid. They are not emotionally vulnerable to your defeats (assuming they have had adequate therapy of their own). They have clear boundaries of time and attention. *They will know if someone is looming far too large in your psyche— and is always a trigger point when you are feeling bad.* (Your partner's troublesome ex might fill this role. It could also be a petty manager at your workplace. Heaven forbid that it is a sibling or an in-law, though in families with unsteady boundaries, that's always possible.)

A caring professional will also know that *this is what you feel right now*, but will feel less acutely in a day, or a month, or at some near point in a future you cannot, at this moment, imagine.

When an emotional pain is fierce, sharp, stinging, it needs expressing. If you don't have a therapist, you can certainly use your journal to write whatever you choose, however you choose. You may also have a friend or family member who will listen without giving you premature advice or cutting you off at the knees with a story of their own.

However, that nonprofessional person may have similar vulnerabilities to yours. They could be over-involved with your well-being and fearful for you, or for themselves. In that case, it will support you and your kind listener to name what you are doing. "I need to vent. This, this, this has happened . . . It would help me if you would listen, but I don't need a solution. I don't need advice. I need very much to express myself, be heard, and have my painful feelings acknowledged."

Venting is quite different from cultivating a dark drama that you return to repeatedly. Or cultivating a grudge, or a longing for revenge. Venting lets difficult feelings get expressed, making space for new experiences.

By naming what you are doing as venting, you are consciously setting some kind of limit to the intensity of the feelings that you are experiencing—even if, at this moment, it seems those uncomfortable emotions will be with you forever. *They will not.* This is what the power of venting allows you to understand.

As legitimate as your feelings are, unless you deliberately stoke them, accelerate them, or keep refueling them, *they will change*.

Hours later, days later—depending on the catalyst—you will allow yourself the small gift of awareness of other, different experiences.

You may find yourself with your hands around a cup of coffee, enjoying the simple warmth, plus the coffee aroma, and the knowledge that after the coffee you and the kids, or you and a friend, or you alone will take a walk, go shopping, watch a series, listen to some music, joke with a neighbor—or just find the energy to face a new day.

In other words, you will still be injured . . . but less so. The sting, though still there, will not be harming you as much. Life is again engaging you. You are living the truth that neither you nor your life is or can be static. It is moving, dynamic. So are you.

(Major griefs are a different matter entirely. Take all the time you need. *And more.* Get and receive all the help you can. *And more.* Be as kind to yourself and others as you have ever been. *And more.*)

46 | Still fragile after all these years

Life is a difficult assignment. We are fragile creatures, expected
to function at high rates of speed, and asked to accomplish great
and small things each day. These daily activities take enormous
amounts of energy. Most things are out of our control. We
are surrounded by danger, frustration, grief, and insanity as
well as love, hope, ecstasy, and wonder. Being fully human is
an exercise in humility, suffering, grace, and great humor.

SARK

The way back to feeling a whole lot better involves connecting more
comfortably with yourself (and therefore others), and regaining your
inborn, never-entirely-lost just-misplaced sense of self-worth and confidence. That's it! Now you have that, you can throw this book away
and go dancing. Or can you?

In situations where anxiety is seriously affecting you, you will
likely feel pushed around by far too much doubt and far too little confidence. That imbalance is uncomfortable enough, but it also undermines your sense of self-worth and makes coping with whatever is in
front of you next to impossible. "I just can't do it." "I'm truly not up
to it." "It's all beyond me." "Get me out of here. Fast."

"Not coping" *and anxiety are inseparable.* Each set of thoughts and feelings feeds off the other. The more the conviction "I'm not coping" dominates your thoughts, the more anxious you are likely to feel.

A distressing degree of not coping affects children's lives. Like many adults, some children will confuse an arbitrary "test" with an assessment of their worth. By twelve, innumerable children feel like enough of a failure to say, "I'm not good at anything," as one heart-breakingly lovely kid said to me recently, because they are not crossing the school hall stage to receive accolades from the principal. This should not determine our sense of self. It does, though.

It's not correct that we will all do better with a "bit of healthy competition." That may work for some, but not when it's attached to a crude binary of one winner and many "also rans." Nor when there is any danger that your very sense of self-worth is tied to achievement. And the fickle nature of other people's judgments, over which you have little or no control.

Rosemary Michalowski is the principal of a Rudolf Steiner (Waldorf) school. She strongly feels that, contrary to mainstream opinion, "A school system that avoids competition and comparison helps young people to have real confidence in their ability to learn."

She continues, "At our school, we actively avoid the use of rewards and punishments. Instead, we foster an attitude where learning is seen as a joy, a rewarding experience in itself. The creative arts enrich the learning as a vibrant 'through-line' bringing to life every facet of learning, not an add-on. A school where deep engagement with learning is actively nurtured helps young people to be genuinely at ease with themselves and their achievements. At the same time, they are in their healthy 'stretch zone'—feeling challenged, but without anxiety about results and rankings. They are learning how to learn. To be 'at ease with ourselves and our environment' is the ideal."

When your mind tightens with anxiety—feeling the pressure—it produces physical tension and creates stress. You know that. You feel it. You may dread it. When you are unafraid (of how you are performing, how you will be judged), you are more likely at any age to throw yourself into the activity and be absorbed by it. That's the wonderful experience that writer and psychologist Mihaly Csikszentmihalyi identifies as *flow* and discusses in his book of the same name. Self-consciousness falls away. Experience comes to the fore.

This freedom from self-consciousness and the merciless opinions of the Inner Critic—as well as external judges—means that you "cope" without judging. Physical and sensual experiences can take you to the same place, although versions of performance anxiety can come in there, too. "Flow" experiences grow out of the freedoms of childhood if a child has had that.

Rosemary again: "Allowing young children time and space to really be children is vital. At our school, children are allowed to play in a way that is entirely self-directed, creative and driven by their own imaginations. They play indoors, they play outdoors, and they are entirely in their element. An immersive experience of creative play in childhood generates a sense of deep happiness that is enriching for the years ahead. Ironically, it is often children and adults in so-called advanced nations who are most caught up in competitive, judgmental anxiety, and least free to be in the flow, to play. (Finland seems to be a rare exception.)"

Play, creativity, pleasure: these are indispensable for genuine "living in the moment," which puts anxiety back in its place.

47 | Positive visualizations can be profound

*We must be learning if we are to feel fully alive, and when life,
or love, becomes too predictable and it seems like there is little
left to learn, we become restless—a protest, perhaps, of the
plastic brain when it can no longer perform its essential task.*

NORMAN DOIDGE

Your mind is more than your brain. Your "self" is more than your
mind. For all that, brain health supports your whole being. And the
discoveries made about the brain in the last couple of decades are at
least as exciting as anyone landing on the moon. And far more relevant
to most of us.

It's the neuroscientists who have shown conclusively that *conditioned
habits of behavior and attitude can be changed*. If you are at all afraid that you
are stuck with responses that harm or limit you, there's a whole world
of new understanding that however young or old you are, you can wake
up new, healthier patterns not just of thinking, but of feeling and responding. I love that. I love that this is evidence-based science. I love
that these changes can be tracked as well as felt. I love that neuroscience
can relieve anxiety and help us change our outlook for the better.

The essential task of the brain is to learn new things. Repeating the "same old, same old" stultifies the brain. So does withdrawing from trying anything new, stimulating, or "a bit too hard." With a new challenge the brain wakes up—if your mind, feelings, and power to choose will allow that.

We live in social and cultural environments where pushing ourselves, regardless of any cost to quality of life, is strongly associated with making money and gaining status in other people's eyes. Learning for its own wondrous sake, or to make our inner lives as well as our outer lives richer, is trivialized. So is learning from the richness of lived experience, and the world of nature all around us.

The intense superficiality that drives so much popular entertainment can numb us, make us less questioning and more compliant. As we move from one private or public situation to another, we can absorb ceaseless stimulation that agitates but fails in any true sense to stimulate us—or wake us up.

In traditional cultures a high degree of sensory alertness to the outer physical environment was necessary for survival. Those of us who are anxious are often highly alert. I know I sometimes feel that my emotional and activist antennae are permanently and unhealthily "up." Through the news and social media, I can feel drawn to this situation of need and that one, appalled especially by the suffering that could so easily be avoided in a kinder, more just world.

We may all need to ask, *alert about what?* How is this helping us, or anyone else, if it also drains us emotionally? How can we be effective when our focus is on all that is wrong, rather than where we can shift some element of collective experience—as well as our own personal "taking in" of the wider world?

At every moment, we are noticing—and not noticing. We are open to these stimuli—not to those. We are focusing here—and unconsciously withdrawing our focus there. All of this shapes what we imprint through the faculties of consciousness and memory.

You and I create memories where we are most attentive. From middle childhood onward, your brain needs you to pay close attention if you are to learn something new, surprising, substantial, or invigorating. That kind of learning experience "turns on" the brain positively.

"Paying attention" is your choice, both as an action and in terms of where your attention "lands." You don't have to formally practice mindfulness meditation to take a little more awareness or consciousness into your day.

"You" can make positive choices. "You" can decide less of that, more of this.

As the focus of your attention changes, feelings will change with it.

Long before I had even heard the word "neuroplasticity," I used positive visualizations in my own life and often in my work with others. This wakes up our natural self-healing. It also stimulates our creativity—essential to feeling alive. But it is neuroscience that lets us know that, in the words of renowned Canadian psychiatrist and psychoanalyst Norman Doidge, writing in *The Brain's Way of Healing*, "Visualization activates the same neurons that are activated when we have the real experiences, visualizing negative experiences or memories triggers all the negative emotional reactions that we had with the original experience—wiring them more deeply into our brains."

That makes it vital to self-care *to notice what you are wiring more deeply into your precious brain. Noticing* is essential to how you will exercise choice. But what's also wondrous for those of us eager to be more robust and less anxious is that remembering and visualizing positive experiences likewise "activates many of the same sensory, motor, emotional, and cognitive circuits that fired during the 'real' pleasant experience," as Dr. Doidge notes.

Hypnotists have known this forever. "See yourself in a beautiful place . . . you are undisturbed by any worries . . . your whole body is trusting and relaxed . . ." Even a very anxious person will find themselves relaxing.

**It's an astonishing thing to discover that brain scans prove
that visualizing yourself moving through a challenging
scenario calmly and positively develops the same changes in
the brain as doing the same action physically and in real time.**

Positive visualizations are immensely reassuring for children, too—maybe even more so if they are lucky enough still to live in the world of story. Imagination can bring children fears. It can also make the inner world a place of creative adventure and excitement.

You can create visualizations together, keeping them simple and always grounding them in everyday experiences, while also bringing in qualities of magic that children universally understand.

TRY THIS
Close your eyes. You may want to rest your palms against your eyes. Simply recall a place where you have felt happy, well and at ease. Let

yourself be in that place. You have all the time in the world. Nothing and no one needs you right now. Enjoy noticing new details, sensory impressions. Take that into your body as you *relax* in this present moment. Come back to everyday awareness only when you have had enough, knowing you are inwardly nourished and refreshed, *thanks to your own self.*

TRY THIS

See yourself in a complex or demanding situation responding with detachment rather than anxiety or anger. Walk through a familiar scenario in your mind that may usually cause you stress. As you do so, try saying: "This is happening outside me, not inside." *The power to detach and not react is key here.* Habits of reaction run deep. Your teenager says this, you say that. And off you both go, with nothing positive achieved. Or maybe it's a sibling or an aged parent with whom you have a complicated history, strongly affected by childhood memories. When you don't play the expected part in the exchanges, those interactions will change in character from tense to more neutral. Watch out for defensiveness. Know *you can soften your own reactiveness.*

TRY THIS

If you can record these longer instructions on your phone, all the better. This is a brief guided meditation to prepare you for any situation that may cause you anxiety or where you feel inadequately prepared.

Close your eyes. You may want to rest your palms against your eyes. Take as much time as you want to feel a sense of positive anticipation. Let that help you relax. If any anxieties intrude, know this is not "their" time; it's yours. Visualize whatever situation you are preparing for. See yourself arriving at the place, the room, the chair where you will be sitting. Imagine these details if you don't yet know. You are rehearsing, walking yourself forward. *It can only go well.*

Notice that you have a backpack that's small and unobtrusive. It has within it any strengths you might need. It's as light as a feather but you slip it off your shoulders to hold it near your belly and your heart. Your posture matters. You are sitting or standing strong, with no tension or stress registering on your face or in your body. Your face is relaxed. So is your throat, shoulders, trunk, arms, hands. Your creativity is switched on. You trust it.

Slowly walk yourself through the scenario where you want to do well. Perhaps it's meeting new people. *You can expect them to like you. You can expect to find something to say as you show an interest in them and in putting them at ease.* Perhaps it's speaking up at a meeting. *You can find the strength you need in your magical backpack.* Perhaps it's having that difficult conversation with a loved one. You see yourself listening carefully, letting go of any defensiveness or anger, and meeting them more than halfway, valuing closeness above "being right."

Before you leave this imagined scene, ask yourself, "Is there anything else I need to notice? Is there a strength in my backpack that I have not yet used? How does it feel now, right now, to have walked through this situation so smoothly? That's me, handling things in the way I want to."

When there are no more questions to be asked, let yourself be aware again of where you are sitting, of where your body is held by your chair, of your feelings of confidence, curiosity—and what else?

Just in your own time, come back to your room and jot down your impressions: what you noticed, what the experience felt like, when or whether you would like to do it again.

This guidance is an example only. Your own creativity will work for you. *Let yourself know what challenge is troubling you. Name that.* Be as precise as you can be. Then write your own positive visualization. This can include whatever you would like to happen. Or what a braver, wiser person than you believe yourself to be might achieve. Or how someone would handle the experience who has the confidence or social skills you most envy. (Turning envy into inspiration is empowering.)

You are a whole self. You have inner resources to draw on at any time, and at all times. You have neurons that will "fire" delightedly when, as Dr. Doidge urges, you try something new, finding out more about your own most positive depths.

48 | Thinking aloud on the page

"How do I know what I think until I hear what I'm saying—or see what I'm writing?"

No machine will ever rival the "unexpectedness" of human consciousness. No machine will ever reach into the collective unconscious, either. Or dip into soul. You don't need to have any formal beliefs to "let the soul speak." Something instinctive within us responds to that permission: "Give voice to the soul, to the wisdom within me, to the depths untouched by anxiety."

"Speaking from your deeper self" has strong similarities with free associating—often part of talk therapies—and with free writing, easily done in your notebook or journal.

Thinking or speaking aloud on the page has many advantages. You are entirely in charge of time and place. Plus, it leads not just to insights but to greater self-trust as you discover how "getting your thoughts down" can bring you the gifts of fresh inspiration. This is particularly moving when it emerges from your own mind and as a treasure from your own lived experience. (Have you ever heard yourself saying something unexpected—and surprisingly helpful? Maybe you even asked yourself with a touch of pride, "Where did that come from?")

This is a universally available version of "thinking aloud" that draws on spontaneity and curiosity, on the mysterious riches of our collective unconscious, rather than offering a familiar, ready-made (or much-repeated or stale) *opinion.*

There is tremendous value in freeing the mind from "stuck thoughts," and making room for what's self-supporting and new. Or for questioning any assumptions that limit you. Or for growing your faculties of awareness, appreciation, praise, and gratitude. Your journal can also be a place to vent, grieve, be unreasonable. And to stand back to ask: *"Where are my thoughts taking me? Is that the direction I am choosing? Is there another way?"*

Such questions are sustaining even when there are no satisfying "answers." Asking the questions is empowering. So is living them. To discover something new emerging from your own mind, self-consciousness needs to take a back seat. So does judgment.

> **When your thoughts are obsessive or self-harming, also write them down. If you don't want others to see them, you can destroy the page or pages immediately, so be fearless. Don't argue with them. Don't try to justify them. Instead, ask yourself those same questions I used above.** *Where are my thoughts taking me? Is that the direction I am choosing? Is there another way?* **And also,** *what small change would bring me greater self-trust? And peace?*

Journaling is an act of self-care that brings insight to the mind and release to your whole self. There's an ancient relationship in writing of releasing and discovering. Enjoy that.

49 | Ways of understanding

Perhaps the last thing you want to do is look closely at what causes you most anxiety. Or maybe you know those causes all too well? The question then becomes what you can do to bring those catalysts down to size, ensuring they don't limit your life further.

Very little can change until you identify what situations or fears disempower you. And as with the exposure therapy that is commonly used for OCD, choice can be restored as you slowly and self-respectfully meet your challenges, monitoring your anxiety rather than being ruled by it.

TRY THIS

Whether you have OCD or any traces of it (as I have), consider if any of these steps taken from the principles of exposure therapy are worth exploring. Be your own researcher and best supporter.

1. Identify in your journal or with a trusted friend or counselor the situations or interactions that most routinely cause you to feel

overwhelmed or inadequate. They may also be the situations you most want to avoid. Don't judge, just list them.

2. If any of those situations causes you harm or endangers you, seek immediate professional help. This exercise is about becoming more open where you would like to be, but anxiety is holding you back.

3. Start with a fear or anxiety that's "not too bad." Write down how your life will be better when this no longer makes you anxious. *Identify the immediate benefits.* ("I want to be able to speak to new people without worrying what they think of me." "I want to look at myself in the mirror and feel good about myself." "It would be great if I was far less irritable when I'm agitated. I want easy good humor." "I'd enjoy life far more if I could do things I enjoy whether or not I am good at them.")

4. Set up a timetable for the gradual steps you will take in re-empowering yourself. ("Week one, I will . . . ; week two, I can . . . ; weeks three and four, I'm going to . . .")

5. If there are setbacks, so what? Just extend your time frame. *You are in charge.*

6. If your anxiety increases rather than shrinks, take smaller steps. *And get help. This is an exercise in facing your fears—with professional support whenever that is needed.*

Talk therapy can often effectively shift the story you are consciously or unconsciously telling yourself. As I write this, I am remembering a well-known actor I worked with in therapy some years ago. He had almost nightly dreams where he would turn up to an audition or for an opening or closing night, and a lifetime of hard work would dissolve into meaninglessness. His mouth would be dry. His memory would be blank. He would be wearing the wrong clothes or turning up at the wrong theater.

Because their work is so unavoidably "out there," an actor is unusually vulnerable when their anxieties become preoccupying or overwhelming. It was obvious to Teddy (not his real name) that his career was at risk. And that identifying and facing his fears was critical to continuing the work he loved. But what were those fears? And why now, when things were going pretty well for him?

Teddy chose to write down his dreams in some detail, looking for ways that anxiety was perhaps trying to protect him. He wanted to understand the story of "wrongness." *At the same time, he asked his agent to increase rather than back away from opportunities for work.* In a way that might have seemed counterintuitive, he encouraged himself to try out for roles that extended his range, even those he was very unlikely to get.

Withdrawing from situations that make you feel more than usually anxious is seldom helpful. (Again, though, DO NOT EVER EXPOSE YOURSELF TO ABUSE, HARM, DISRESPECT, OR HURT.) Teddy's counterintuitive boldness grew into greater confidence, not as an "actor" but in himself. Rather than "shrinking," he was expanding emotionally.

Turning up in the wrong place, wearing the wrong clothes (or no clothes), or not learning or looking "the part" is a dream that happens in various forms to many of us who are not actors. Or are we?

In the most authentic life, you play a number of roles. Some will fit you, some less so. Some demands you can face with equanimity, some not.

When you are looking at what causes you most anxiety, and where you have least confidence, *check carefully what you are expecting of yourself.*

Check, too, what you are telling yourself about the situation—and whether that internal narrative is encouraging and supporting you or is making your anxiety worse.

Children with school avoidance issues, for example, need to be helped to face school, and their fears, through small steps that rebuild self-confidence not in the direction of school only, but more generally. *A particularly challenging situation is always part of a bigger picture.*

Teddy's anxiety was in part a product of getting older in a cruelly ageist profession. Was he still a "good fit" for what producers or directors wanted? He felt their power acutely, so taking back his power through *voluntarily increasing his risk-taking* was a big act of self-respect and trust. And a bold way of working with time, rather than letting the anxieties of aging (illness and death) defeat him.

Each of us will play, as the famous line from Shakespeare's *As You Like It* says, many parts. That short speech ends lugubriously: "Last scene of all, / That ends this strange eventful history, / Is second childishness and mere oblivion; / Sans teeth, sans eyes, sans taste, sans everything."

Can we assume Shakespeare wrote this as a very young man, with "oblivion" as well as toothlessness seeming a long way off? In the four hundred years since, we have more choices than Shakespeare with his genius could have dreamed of. Just like for Shakespeare, though, time is not on our side. Identifying our fears, meeting them with curiosity and at least a little trust, brings us time. Plus, ideally, a little more choice in how we use it.

50 | Checking my checking

Perhaps like you, I know very few people with intrusive anxiety who don't have some traces of OCD, especially when they are under greater pressure than usual. That's my experience, certainly. And as I spoke to people while writing this book, it became ever clearer to me that obsessive thinking, with or without compulsive actions, is on the rise. It is a major robber of peace of mind. It is also horribly undermining of one's sense of self. ("If I can't trust myself to have carried out my compulsive behaviors well enough, how can I trust myself?")

My own most frequent irrational (obsessive) anxiety is around the locking of doors: Have I locked my doors, is my house safe? (*Is my life safe? Is my family safe?*) This is certainly a trust issue, a rescuing issue, a keeping-everyone-secure issue.

From a psychoanalytic perspective, the particularities of our obsessive anxieties almost always tell a meaningful story, and my situation is no exception.

I could explain my lock/security worries by telling you that as a single parent of two children I felt wholly responsible for their well-being.

They had and have a father. I have at least some faith in the spiritual strengths we can only guess at. Nonetheless, providing my children and myself with a home where we would feel safe was more than a primary goal for me. It was an obsession. My inner safety depended upon my capacity to do this—and to do it independently.

More than that, because my own mother had died of cancer while I was still a young child (aged eight), it was my greatest fear and dread that I would leave my children abandoned and motherless. In other words, not just lacking the secure home that I must provide, but without a mother—a trauma that I have grown "around" without ever fully recovering from it.

I see now that I was unusually determined from a very early age to do whatever it took—however many extra jobs it took—to provide myself with a home of my own. I didn't expect a husband or partner to provide this for me. Nor did that ever happen. I bought a tiny flat in London's then-unfashionable North Kensington in my twenties. Two years later, I bought a house that wasn't much bigger in East London. However, when I came to Australia in my mid-thirties, and had my children—born just over a year apart—that drive around house/ home, providing/caring became more complex, and a greater source of anxiety.

Several things happened at once. My children's father and I separated. I had breast cancer. There was serious acrimony over property. I feared losing my house / our home. My anxiety levels were at an all-time high, unsurprisingly, and I developed what it took me a while to recognize as OCD around locks and locking, a literalization of my efforts to protect the children, and myself. Locking up became a ritual of security that I could not entirely trust, any more than I could entirely trust my power to keep the children safe from all dangers—including their mother not staying alive.

The irony is that someone did once break into that house and it was in broad daylight. I was working in my attic office at the top of the house when I heard a noise downstairs.

The children were at school, so I knew it wasn't them making sounds. Without hesitating, and I think at the time without fear, I went to the stairs and, as I came down, saw a man in our large kitchen area. Totally instinctively—as I told my sister later—I channeled our maternal grandmother, a woman of authority and courage, and said, loudly, "How dare you come into this house? Get out now. Get out straightaway." And he did! Thank heaven. The police told me later that I had been foolhardy, not courageous. Or perhaps I was just lucky.

These days, my children are no longer children and I feel better and far safer within myself. There are times, though, when I will still need to check and recheck several times that I have locked up my house (and sometimes my car).

That means overriding my clear memories of locking "just in case." It may mean driving home again from several kilometers away. It may mean walking back not once but more than once.

Such compulsions are irrational. Sufferers know that. They are also wildly intrusive. Sufferers know that, too. Many of us find methods to counteract our fears, or to reassure ourselves with conscious measures like mindfully touching the locked door and saying, "I am fully aware this door is locked."

It is also possible these days to get a photo using your phone. "Anchoring" the reassurance through some form of intense focus—however fleeting—can soothe the anxieties that are inaccessible to "common sense" (or other people's irritated incredulity).

People suffering from OCD urgently need specialist medical treatment that reduces rather than worsens their anxiety while they go through the rigors of exposure therapy. They/you cannot do this alone. Sufferers who may be more in the generalized anxiety camp, as I was or am, may benefit from my best, hard-won discovery.

When I notice obsessive thoughts pushing their way to the front of my consciousness and demanding attention, *I now know that my general anxiety needs attention.* In other words, I use my bursts of obsessive-compulsive worry about security and safety, and how adequately I am caring for others as a barometer. I am pushed to ask: What am I not paying attention to; where have I neglected to keep myself safe in some significant way?

It may seem paradoxical to "use" a very uncomfortable pattern in this way. But it strengthens me. I don't expect ever to entirely lose my worries about locking, safety, *heightened responsibility for the care of others.* There's merit there. What I can do is tame the extreme manifestations of those thought habits. Once again, more compassionate self-care provides the tools.

51 | Challenge hopeless

"Hopeless" is a wretched state of mind. It is also a powerfully condemning way to think about yourself—or anyone else. When applied to yourself, it speaks of a tragic loss of faith. *No one is hopeless.* When applied to others, it speaks of a profound lack of respect.

To call someone "hopeless" is to set yourself up as judge, jury, and executioner. To call yourself hopeless is to betray a whole-self perspective that assures you that however hard things may seem, you have resources; you have values, goals, good intentions, and feelings—and the capacity to access them.

"Hopeless" may seem to belong more in the realm of depression than of anxiety. Yet because anxiety—like depression—reduces your capacity to think creatively and assertively, feelings of hopelessness as well as helplessness affect many people.

William Styron is the author of a famous novel called *Sophie's Choice*. He has also written a memoir of his suffering from depression that seems relevant for anxiety sufferers also. In *Darkness Visible: A Memoir of Madness*, he writes, "It is hopelessness even more than pain that crushes the soul. So the decision-making of everyday life involves not, as in normal affairs, shifting from one annoying situation to another less annoying—or from discomfort to relative comfort, or from boredom to activity—but moving from pain to pain."

Moving from pain to pain. This phrase breaks my heart. And it makes me angry that so many suffer. The particular pain of hopelessness is sly, pervasive, and destructive. What it takes from you is the memory of the countless situations you have already met positively.

When you're flooded with dread, or your phobias or OCD are shaping your days, or you are lying awake at 3 a.m. reviewing all the things that might have and certainly will go wrong, you need an antidote that is powerful enough to meet what might otherwise crush you.

Shifting yourself away from all-or-nothing thinking matters here. The big "H" words (hate, hopeless, helpless) *can never support you.* It may seem counterintuitive to say to yourself in these moments, "Hopeless is what I feel . . . it is totally NOT who I am."

But that is true. It is not even a scrap of who you are.

**If you take nothing else from this book, please
vow that you will eliminate "hate," "hopeless" and
"helpless" from your thinking, your labeling, and even
your feelings about yourself—and anyone else.**

Will that "cure" your anxiety, or treat it? It may. It will certainly go far in restoring self-respect, self-trust, and inner security. Hopeless? I think not.

52 | Abandonment anxiety

When you feel more than desperate, more than anxious, and that your well-being depends on the presence of one particular person, this is a primal agony that traces back to the earliest days of your existence. It is one of the greatest fears that you can experience.

If you know a fear of abandonment is your particular vulnerability, and that your situation with a loved person is fragile, it is essential to understand also that a more realistic danger is, in fact, *abandoning yourself.*

No fear, however urgent, describes all of who you are.
You are a whole self.
You have resources to make your inner and outer worlds richer.
You belong to life; we all do.

The abandonment anxiety you feel is not happening in a vacuum. It is a common tendency in twenty-first-century life to depend intensely on a single person who "should" meet all your needs. And to feel desolate when that person is in your life but is not fulfilling your hopes. Or isn't in your life at all, except as the focus of your yearning. (That's the plot of every rom-com, however good or bad.)

You might also live in a town or city where too few people know you as anything more than a colleague, neighbor, or acquaintance. Or maybe you are mostly acknowledged in your multiple roles: office manager, Eric's boss, the twins' parent, kids' baseball coach, the person who can be relied upon always to turn up—except for herself.

Under those very familiar circumstances, your "one and only person"—real or desired—can easily have more power over your inner stability than you or they would want.

There is no easy fix. Shifting your center of gravity from outside to inside yourself takes will and a ton of courage. If you are in a relationship with a flawed, complex human being—much like you or me—this gravity shift need not and should not necessitate pushing the other person far away. It does, however, ask you to look honestly at what your unconscious expectations are—and where they are out of sync with what you know is healthy. There's a lot in this book about self-trust. And about compassion. What I write less explicitly about is self-love. I should be braver.

> **Self-love cannot coexist with disparaging thoughts about yourself. Self-love will not be present when you cannot trust your own self to "save your life."**

Self-love does not mean self-absorption. On the contrary, it means appreciating the unique gift of life that you have, the whole self that you are, with gifts as well as challenges all contributing to the person that you are today and are becoming tomorrow. In *The Ikigai Journey*, one of the Spanish writers, Francesc Miralles, names as one of his "crucial decisions" the following: "Never again to beg for anyone's affection. If someone decides to distance themselves from me, I let them go and stop fighting for their attention, however much we may have shared previously. Within this category, I would include freeing myself from the obligation to always be friendly. It is no big deal if somebody can't stand you—you cannot please everybody."

Francesc—the author of many novels and nonfiction works—is a far tougher person than I am! And perhaps than you are? However, when you know your abandonment issues are reaching desperation levels, it is essential to get professional help to address those terrifying feelings.

They are central to your anxiety, to the way it influences your thinking, muddles your judgment, and revs up your fears. When you most fear abandonment, you urgently need self-understanding, compassion, and tenderness to get you back onto solid ground within yourself—the best possible place from which to reach out to receive another's affection. And give it.

(If someone plays with your feelings or seems to get any kind of kick out of your vulnerability, *that is abuse.* Professional help is needed. No halfway healthy person ever wants to increase the suffering of another human being, in any way, or in any form.)

53 | Keep space for the beautiful

I consider the people I most love my human trees—people
firmly rooted in a foundation of moral beauty, relentlessly
reaching for the light, bent into their particular beloved shape
by the demands and traumas of their particular lives.

MARIA POPOVA

I was recently at an exciting exhibition of contemporary art with two friends. One was enchanted with the exhibition, as I was. The other was less intrigued. Art, he said, was not his thing. Nonetheless, he asked me what I thought was a most intriguing question.

Many of the exhibits related to the natural environment, as well as built-up environments. "How was it different," he asked, "to look at these representations rather than at the environments themselves—particularly the natural environments, which are so endlessly wondrous?" (My friend is a surfer as well as a scientist.)

I would be interested to know what your response might be to his question. Mine was that in an art gallery we see creative responses to the subject matter—the world around us, in this instance—through multiple perspectives. In other words, we are seeing the world we think we know, *and* glimpsing an incredible diversity of views.

That affirms your own capacities to switch, change, *grow a new point of view.* Knowing, too, that this view may change—and why not? It also brings you more securely into the limitlessness of human experience. To see the world as another sees it is a great gift that drives our interest well beyond art. That's wondrous in itself.

The constant changes within nature, the paradoxical predictability of change, has its echoes in you. Anxiety can make change difficult. But an experiential recognition of "Ah, I see that differently now" is liberating.

When you are enjoying nature at her freest, or you are walking on a busy city street aware of the air, the weather, the birds, the occasional tree, the built environment and crowds of people, you are experiencing something through your own perceptions and vision.

All art forms, including writing, let you expand your way of seeing. Sometimes, this is what you are seeing on the outside—like you do in the street. Just as often, art can jolt you enough to see something differently—or more appreciatively—that could be on the outside, but it's *your inner experience that's changing.*

Does this mean you will automatically experience the beautiful, the wondrous, the awesome more intensely? I'm not sure. What I do know is that will happen only when you willingly make space for it. Only when you welcome it.

54 | Best medicine

May the relief of laughter rinse through your soul.
JOHN O'DONOHUE

Pleasure, curiosity, adventure, engagement, and connection with other people are all the "best medicine." In fact, the loss of pleasure in everyday living is one of the cruelest effects of depression—and also chronic or acute anxiety. Anxiety affects your power to initiate as well as organize. Pleasant daily tasks can become "too much." Ordinary socializing can lose its sheen even when some company could lift mood and spirits. This reluctance may be due to a lack of energy. It may also come from heightened self-consciousness and a dread you are being judged harshly.

If anxiety or depression is bringing you down right now, it will be hard to rally and look outward. The emergency measures in part two may help best. Yet, even then, at least try some of these simple measures, especially anything that gets your body moving forward, perhaps your emotions with it, and your spirits upward.

TRY THIS

- First thing in the morning, go outside and turn your face up to the sky. Is it raining? Snowing? Bright sunshine? Cloudy? Soft air or a gale wind? Enjoy the sensations of *this moment* without rushing. Let seasonal changes remind you that *nothing is permanent*, even the hardest of mind states. (If you have little children, get them to do this with you. They will love it!)

- Check if there are pleasures other people enjoy that you envy, or wish, "If only . . ." Or, are there pleasures you once enjoyed that feel lost to you now? *Take some risks.* Keep the idea of nonjudgmental *experimenting* front of mind.

- Find a people-friendly activity where nothing particularly personal is asked of you: *anything where kindness is present* from community gardening to volunteering, a class, a public talk on something that matters. My years of gospel singing were brilliant for this. In fact, a love of music, chant, movement is your birthright. Music reaches beyond words. *The body hears it.* Your entire self will benefit.

55 | In your own hands

When I'm taking action, I don't feel like I am
helpless . . . and that things are hopeless, because then I
feel like . . . I'm doing everything I can. And that gives
me very much hope, especially to see all the other people all
around the world, the activists, who are taking action and
who are fighting for their present and for their future.

GRETA THUNBERG

There's a low (and sometimes rising) hum of anxiety in most people's lives from whatever aspects of life they can't control. Some of these will be very personal—like vile views about our race, perhaps, or our gender, or our choices of who and how we will love. Maybe we lack the privileges of birth or status that seem to give others a free pass? Maybe we are peacemakers in a world obsessed with guns and war and violence?

Maybe we are noticing with horror the vast and widening gaps between the obscenely wealthy and the deliberately impoverished, destroying fair and equitable access to basic housing, education, and health care? Or that differences in life expectancy between rich and poor can be as much as fifteen years in a "lucky" nation?

In recent times, our awesome planet has been kicking back against centuries of greed-driven, gross mismanagement. I am writing these words in Australia where the many First Nations peoples of this continent can correctly claim to be the longest-surviving cultures in the world, stretching back 60,000 or even 80,000 years. They must weep about the madness of a mere 200 years.

Yet with the unchecked escalation of greenhouse gases in the atmosphere, plus unchecked plundering of the land and its resources, "once-in-a-century" droughts, floods, and fires are with us right now, sometimes only weeks apart as homes are burned or washed away, whole towns wrecked, lives lost. And still the fossil fuel global corporations have a seat at the highest tables in the land, as they do in all "advanced" economies, while the most drastic effects of climate change (as well as pandemics) are suffered by the poorest. *Who wouldn't be anxious?* Who wouldn't wake at night occasionally or often asking, as the Peter, Paul and Mary song goes, "When will they ever learn? When will they *ever* learn?"

In Milan, Italy, in 2021, climate activist and global leader Greta Thunberg said, "We can no longer let the people in power decide what is politically possible. We can no longer let the people in power decide what hope is. Hope is not passive. Hope is not blah, blah, blah. Hope is telling the truth. Hope is taking action. And hope always comes from the people."

"Eco-anxiety" is real. It is daunting. It is confusing. It is terribly frightening. Especially when those denying climate change or trivializing it are everywhere in global media. No wonder people increasingly turn to video games, or binge-watching on Netflix or similar apps where even with apocalyptic series, they can pick up the remote to switch the series off as well as on, and comfort themselves with the thought that it is all fiction.

But the central conviction driving my work generally—and this book—is that each of us is unconditionally part of a whole universe. Most of us barely understand the extent of our interdependence. Yet it is a truth. *The part that each of us plays, however modest, however unnoticed, matters.* Our lives—yours and mine—matter. The empowerment that comes from bringing meaning to those efforts and to our whole existence profoundly matters.

It is an outrageous lie that we can do nothing about our world . . . or our anxieties about the world and ourselves. It is a lie. We can choose to be manipulated into despair, indifference, or nihilism. But that will make it far harder to meet candidly and courageously the anxieties that are closest to home, that reverberate in our bodies, our emotions, our souls.

TRY THIS

Take heart from your smallest personal actions that reflect greater hope—and the actions hope inspires. *Sometimes all you can do is begin, slowly, to take better care of yourself.* Yet, this is itself a gift to the world around you. Your small shifts inevitably affect the world of which you are a part, as well as your own self. As you feel stronger, your engagement with others and the wider world will reflect that, quite naturally.

That's what self-therapy is: taking compassionate, self-respectful, creative, thoughtful action that will shift the way you see yourself, your resources, the sacredness of your unique existence, alongside so many others playing their part. It will also shift the way you see the world and "power."

That wisdom, at the very least, is in your own hands.

56 | Coming to terms with the way things are

"Coming to terms with the way things are" should not be confused with passive resignation, helplessness, or despair. Nor is it quite the same as the Serenity Prayer, which in a 1933 version attributed to Winnifred Crane Wygal went: "Father, give us courage to change what must be altered, serenity to accept what cannot be helped, and the insight to know the one from the other."

The Serenity Prayer is a call to truth, which is a quality that courage both demands and gives. But "coming to terms with the way things are" may ask of you an inner fortitude and self-valuing of a very particular kind. This will be harder still to achieve if you want nothing more than to hide or run away. Or worse.

Can you think of times in your life when you have fought desperately against a reality that seems unbearable? When you have found yourself saying, "Surely not?"

Your lover or partner has abandoned you. A colleague has betrayed you. You are dangerously ill, physically or mentally. You have been told that it is impossible for you to have the baby you longed for. You are dying, far too young. One of your children is living a life that endangers them. Perhaps you have lost your faith in the God you trusted to be faithful to you? Or maybe what you have lost is a sense of meaning, purpose, direction?

It could also be that you find yourself without a home, a victim of an economic system that has no regard for human dignity.

Those crossroad moments come in every life—perhaps not always as dramatically, but to the person experiencing them the suffering feels profound.

I doubt that many of us would say we're ready to bear the anguish they bring with them. At such times, it feels as though you can't go back and, simultaneously, that there is no way forward. Yet life does not stand still.

The very nature of existence is ever-changing and dynamic, however stuck you feel.

Fighting against the way things are, you will be piling suffering onto pain, and pain onto suffering. In the depths of your soul, you might cry, "I can't go on like this." Or, "This is unendurable." Or, "This is more than I can bear." The stress of such times is harrowing. It feels unendurable. While it possesses you, the rest of your existence will feel like a blank. And yet we do endure, of course.

Whatever the source of your anguish, you cannot begin to heal its effects until you stop fighting against it. "Healing" may strike you as an odd word to use here. *Yet healing means finding the courage to accept what cannot be helped or changed.* It means accepting the devastation not as a failure, not as a judgment, not as a particular torment for you but, rather, as a part of this mysteriously complex process we call human existence.

Good and bad things happen to good and bad people. It is not that you or I have been singled out: it is that grief, disappointment, illness, betrayal, death—especially illness and death—will come in some form to all of us, without exception.

Not for a moment do I assume that accepting an "impossible" reality is easy. Even to grasp it as a possibility may seem like several bridges too far. The idea of accepting a totally unwelcome situation rather than fighting against it may arouse in you, as it has in me, fears greater than anything you have previously experienced. This may be all your dreads come true. One young man, Evan, whose beloved partner was killed in a car crash, said to me, "This isn't a nightmare. There is no waking up."

Your envy of people who seem to have an untroubled life may be strong at such times. ("Why me . . . ?" "Why us?") Your feelings of inadequacy and inability to cope may be worse than the blow itself. This can be true with the torment of untreated mental illness also.

Devorah is a doctor in her early thirties, the mother of two children, a winner of university prizes and destined for a glittering career. A year ago, she was diagnosed first with a psychotic depression, then with MDD (major depressive disorder), then most recently with bipolar II. Her response? "Anything but this. Give me the worst cancer over this. I don't know if the people I work with would really feel embarrassed if they find out . . . or if it's just me. But I prefer to put on a fake face for work and get through my days without their pity. Or their questions. Or their assumptions that I won't cope and have to be treated like a bomb about to go off."

Neither Evan nor Devorah can easily believe in anything resembling a normal life coming again. Evan's partner was his closest friend, his "favorite person in the whole world." The suddenness of the death was worsened by its randomness.

Devorah's situation is different. She is a doctor, hugely frustrated by the different diagnoses she has received and the inadequate medication that followed each. But she does have access to specialist treatment and the chances are good that the right medication will be found and supportive therapy can get her through the worst of the lasting trauma of the past year.

Nonetheless, however the future looks, living in denial of *how things are* consumes immeasurable amounts of energy. Living in fear of other people's negative reactions, as Devorah does, adds to our pain and cannot lessen it. Some people will react stupidly or thoughtlessly. Some will do much better. We can't change that.

Facing *what is* from the perspective of the whole self, and the truth of a whole life, there will emerge moments of refuge, slivers of comfort. With truth, at least some tension will fall away. The grief or outrage will still be there, but you will find yourself facing forward, rather than backward. You will glimpse solid ground, rather than quicksand. Can any of us ask more of ourselves than that? What's more, for some, there is a degree of social understanding that may not relieve your personal vulnerability, but at least you are not also dealing with others' judgments, as well as your own.

Thomas is a twenty-one-year-old university student studying social economics. Perhaps his level of education and liberal family background make him more relaxed than some might be. I was nonetheless pleased to hear that in his social circles being anxious is completely acceptable. In Thomas's words, "My experience is that a lot of people around my age are accepting and understanding of anxiety."

He's lucky enough not to experience much anxiety around his studies, although he adds, "I think I do worry how people will judge me, though that's more subconscious than a conscious thought. Also, I like to believe I am easy to get to know, though at times I catch myself putting up walls [to prevent others from getting] to know me more deeply. When I experience social anxiety, my go-to method for dealing with it is to explain away the feelings. I may feel others will judge me, but I am also aware it is not something I would even pay attention to if someone else did. If I am anxious, most frequently I'll find myself in bed with a book or playing a video game to unwind. Reading an interesting nonfiction book helps zone out anything else going on and I always enjoy the experience."

There was a tougher period in Thomas's life, and that's where therapy did help. He explains that here.

At the end of my first year, I experienced a long period of depression and so made the decision to start therapy. The main focus was generally related to depression rather than anxiety. This included working on building healthy habits, including getting better sleep and more physical exercise, which I suspect also impacted feelings of anxiety. Therapy encouraged me to be more conscious of depression and anxiety, and taking steps in the moment to counteract those feelings.

With anxiety the biggest takeaway that has been the most useful to me has been just to take a moment and look at the situation from an external perspective. Regularly just thinking about how I would feel about someone else in my situation is enough to build up enough courage to get involved. My anxiety is strongest before participating in a new social situation. Getting past that initial anxiety has been crucial for me and how I experience anxiety.

I don't believe that the anxiety I tend to experience is inevitable. I suspect it is somewhat self-reinforcing where I remember feeling anxious in a similar situation previously, and that memory makes me anxious where I wouldn't otherwise have been. In most day-to-day situations now I am not particularly intruded on by anxiety. Compared to many of my friends, I think I am particularly comfortable in academic situations. I am definitely most impacted by anxiety in situations involving new people. Particularly when trying something involving a new skill.

There was also a situation of moving out of college at the start of COVID. Though the logistics of getting back to my home city with lockdowns did cause some worry, I think in particular it was feeling unable to control the situation. Having organized everything, when thinking about it rationally, I knew it would be fine—but in the moment I wanted to do more to make sure everything went according to plan. Definitely I felt some anxiety from the possibility of something going wrong, but it was the lack of control in the situation that made me particularly anxious.

57 | Peace in real time

It isn't enough to talk about peace, one must believe in it.
And it isn't enough to believe in it. One must work at it.

ELEANOR ROOSEVELT

Essential to our efforts for a kinder, more peaceful world on the "outside" is finding greater equanimity on the inside. This does not mean all your anxiety or fears will miraculously disappear. Some elements of anxiety are helpful to you in keeping you safe or avoiding dangerous recklessness. A "pinch of anxiety" can also stimulate you, get you better prepared for what's to come, put you on your toes. What is not helpful is when anxiety runs riot, or stands up like a rabid dictator shouting orders and disrespecting you.

This entire book supports putting anxiety back in its place and bringing you a far greater sense of your own power to moderate your moods and quieten your fears. However, it is most definitely worth considering which situations, people, and ideas enhance your sense of equanimity and relative peace, and which do not.

For more than two decades I have followed world teacher of peace Thich Nhat Hanh. More than any other teacher I have known, he understood peace not as a noble idea only (though it is that), but as a way of being in the world. *And a way of being inside your own life.*

"Peace" should not be confused with simply avoiding conflict, or with passivity. It takes strength of mind and character to walk peace's path. And to value nonviolent action over any form of violent action (including in our own minds and hearts).

A focus on peace—and seeing yourself as a source of peace—is strengthening for your mind, even or especially when anxiety has taught you how easily peace, and peace of mind, can be disrupted.

Ours is a world with media that thrives on "taking sides," competitiveness, and ceaseless conflict; that trivializes the big issues; that presents violence as "entertainment" even for children.

Surviving all that takes fortitude of a rare kind.

And we want to do better than survive. We want to live—or I do, at least—with passion, appreciation, excitement, curiosity, as well as the ability to be silent and content in our own company. All of that becomes far more likely when we are not lured and distracted by whatever is highlighted on today's Anxiety Menu.

On the spiritual retreats I lead, I invariably share a small prayer adapted from Thich Nhat Hanh's prayers and poetry. It goes like this (and can be repeated as often as you wish, and said as slowly as you wish):

> *As I breathe in, my body calms.*
> *As I breathe out, I am smiling.*
> *Unlimited moments stretch before me.*
> *I vow to see all beings in the light of acceptance and compassion.*

(This vow needs to include seeing *yourself* also "in the light of acceptance and compassion." Often, that's what is most needed.)

58 | Not helpless, not hopeless

During our most recent Christmas period, an unusually stoic friend was confronted with a situation that instantly drained his usual pragmatic equilibrium. What he was left with was fear and panic.

He had news that his adult daughter and her family were in a car crash caused by a drunk driver plowing through a red light and straight into their car. All he knew was that the car was wrecked, the parents and one of the children were in the hospital, and the outlook was serious. My friend is an emergency room doctor. He is used to dealing with disasters in a way most of us are not. But this was different. What's more, in a strange replay, a decade or so earlier when his daughter was a student, she and her mother had been in an eerily similar accident, again on Christmas Day: drunk driver, red light, car wrecked, and the mother and daughter lucky to be alive.

His daughter's luck held this second time, too, if it is possible to say that after two bone-jarring escapes caused by a driver's drunken disregard for other people's lives. For my friend, though, it was a wake-up call in two distinct directions. First, it was an unwelcome reminder of the painful truth that in all our lives there are situations we can't control. Second, the agony of helplessness—being unable to fix, save, rescue, control the outcome—takes any one of us to a level of suffering that's all on its own.

Every person who has stood by the bed of a loved one who is dying long before they "should." Or has a beloved person suffering a catastrophic illness of any kind. Or is enduring the unendurable grieving for someone who has ended their own life, or who is supporting a dear person who has lost their will to live. They will know more than I can describe here.

If one of your inner archetypal figures is a Rescuer, this may be a particular horror. By inner archetypes, I mean an aspect of your self that seems to direct your consciousness, strongly influencing the way you interpret events and the part you should/must/need to play in them. (Perhaps the Inner Critic is also an archetype in a society as judgmental and competitive as ours is.)

The Rescuer is an archetype that's been intense in me since childhood—though it was then the very last idea I could have made conscious. I have spent more than half my life studying the human condition, our challenges, and our potentials for living fully as well as healing. I have done this through immersing myself in the worlds of therapy as a patient and a practitioner, and through even more years of spiritual study across the major faiths.

Writing the books that have absorbed and taught me so much has also been at least as central to my "education" as formal academic studies.

This inner impulse to support others psychologically and spiritually is a way of supporting myself also, and I feel privileged in what I learn and receive from it. Perhaps this same impulse drives my activism in the wider world, too. And it has inspired me to push myself so much further than I could ever have imagined as a girl or younger woman. Yet it has not rescued me from the disabling fears, the anxiety I have, when someone I love is suffering acutely, and I feel again the trauma of helplessness from the past. And it is trauma. It is a loss of certainty that's so acute your world tips on its axis and doesn't again right itself.

I'm tempted to say we have had more than our share of illness and emotional trauma in our family: my family of origin and the family I created. But *more than our share* is not a claim any of us can reasonably make when we also have access to support, a home to live in, people to comfort and inspire us, and some aspects of life that have gone wonderfully well.

So how do I calm that Inner Rescuer now, if I am consumed by anxiety about a loved one?

I remind myself repeatedly of the truth that "rescuing" never depends on one person, one set of circumstances. My child self unconscious could not fathom this. My adult self can, and I must accept it. I pray often. I surround the person I am most worried about with golden healing light, taking the chance that this might possibly affect them more positively than anxious worrying. I inquire what practical help I can give—and do at least that. (Practical help can be far more effective in hard moments than talking.) I accept help from my family and the few closest friends who can tolerate my lack of social energy— never outstanding at the best of times.

As a high priority, I make time to be alone as that has always served me well as a way of restoring myself to myself so that I can be present for those who need me. Temperament comes in here. Extroverts may want lots of engagement; introverts much less so.

I do pay attention to my body because high levels of anxiety affect my skin (rashes), cause headaches and dire sleeplessness, and worsen chronic pain. I do a modest amount of walking and spend time in my courtyard gardens that flourish even when I don't. I read novels and poetry to give my mind a break. (Again, a faithful, self-rescuing habit.) I take medication for pain. I breathe in compassion and breathe it out again, hoping something reaches my soul. I prioritize and enjoy simple practical tasks around the house, while also not worrying much about those same tasks on days when care of the loved one comes first. I eat reasonably well, certainly healthily. I think and write—sometimes intensely. And I listen to wiser friends who remind me that joy, yes joy, not just relief from anxiety, will also always come again.

59 | Tough experiences are never wasted

There are many situations and experiences that I wholeheartedly wish I had avoided. I took risks as a young woman that I see now were reckless, even dangerous. On a recent visit to New Zealand, the country where I was born and grew up, I heard a friend describing some of the risks she had taken, traveling the world alone as a very young woman, as I had done. She was certainly not boasting, and as she and I exchanged glances, she understood, as I do, that a bit more fear would have kept her safer. As it would have done me.

It wasn't that I was unafraid of the risks I was taking. It was really that *I did not see the intrinsic value of my own life.* That's a big statement. It may ring true, though, for you also if anxiety or depression or trauma has lessened your connection to yourself. Or made that precious connection negative and fragile, rather than positive and strong.

Looking at the bigger, more truthful picture of your whole, complex, sometimes contradictory self, you can discover that even your most difficult experiences need not be wasted. *Nor do they determine or predict what's to come*, no matter how grim your expectations are. (*"Everything* I do goes badly" and "I have the worst luck of anyone I know" are two statements you could certainly challenge.)

Attitude and action are the yin and yang here; attitude, though, must take the lead. Until you have that somewhat more generous vision of yourself, I or any other writer could give you a thousand strategies and not much would change fundamentally. Anxiety, anxious depression, OCD, phobias, panic attacks, or difficulties with food, drink, drugs— or other people—would still have disproportionate power in your life. And that's tragic.

> **We live in a world where we are facing collective crises
> on every front. To feel anxious about and within this
> world may be inevitable. What's not inevitable is to lose
> touch with your power to choose awe and kindness and
> laughter and music and silliness and meaning and sensuality.
> Whatever your gender, race, or culture, the fullness of
> life should be yours. Anxiety erodes that. Anxiety may
> even destroy that fullness—and your vitality with it.**

I gave this book the most startling title I could dream up: *Your name is not Anxious.* I wanted to catch your attention from the start because, no matter how fierce controlling anxiety seems to be, you are always more than even your very worst fears. More than your obsessive thoughts. More than those harsh things you may have been saying to yourself. More than your perfectionism. More than your status anxiety. More than your paralyzing social self-consciousness. More than your addictions and unhealthy dependencies. Far more than your panic attacks. Infinitely more than the voice that tells you it's in any way rational to harm yourself.

You are also more than the judgments inside your own mind that you are attributing to other people ("I know they think I am hopeless.") And aren't you also more than the person who feels afraid to enter a room of strangers, or to reveal who you "really are" to someone trying to know you?

Perhaps you believe that ordinary mistakes will mark you forever in the eyes of other people. Or that your sense of inner reality depends on constantly achieving new levels of success.

Your body, too, will be telling stories about your anxious fears. Perhaps this is through chronic sleeplessness, headaches, or a painful back that has no obvious origin. It may be shortness of breath, pain in your guts, or a tension that never seems to let you go.

It may be a conviction that you can't relax without a glass of wine. Or three or four. You may be familiar, too, with a kind of foreboding that even if things are relatively fine today, tomorrow something terrible will happen. And you will have no more power over those events than you do over anxiety.

Foreboding is a state of mind that I have felt, as well as studied. I know it from the inside out. I also know that some of us are far more vulnerable to anxiety than others, and that even the most resilient people will have limits.

In whatever way anxiety manifests in your life, if it is constraining, overwhelming, or flooding you—or "just" pushing its way in when your everyday stresses grow too big to handle—then it is essential to put anxiety back in its place. And to know not just how to do that, but that *you can do that*.

You do that by gaining a bigger, truer view of yourself—as each storyteller in this book demonstrates. This is far richer and more stabilizing than simply thinking more positively. Your patterns/habits of thinking are learned, conditioned, *and not inevitable.* Noticing how you see yourself right now is key to gaining a bigger, kinder view of yourself and *your whole unique and precious life.* While there is so much going on in our crazy world that you can't immediately change for the better, your inner world is another matter entirely.

I treasure this quote from poet-philosopher Pádraig Ó Tuama, who tells us, "In Irish when you talk about emotion, you don't say, 'I am sad.' You would say, 'Sadness is on me.' *Tá brón orm.* And I love that," he continues, "because there's an implication of not identifying yourself with the emotion fully. I am not sad, it's just that sadness is on me for a while. Something else will be on me another time, and that's a good thing to recognize."

How exhilarating that this *different act of describing* offers a way into *feeling different* also.

Observing how you are encouraging and supporting yourself and those around you is self-therapy at its most healing and most effective. It demands attention to yourself. It demands attention to others. We are, oh yes we are, in this life together.

60 | Doing well. Being well.

I want to start with a story—not just because I love stories and treasure our timeless interest in hearing them—but also because in writing this book I discovered that storytelling is so inevitable it has been called "the default position" of the brain. Through story, you can soothe your body. And your mind. You can shift your perceptions of the world.

You and I are constantly telling ourselves stories. Whether or not we are conscious of it, we are rerunning scenarios, putting our own stamp on them, lifting our spirits with them, or dashing hope. The stories we tell ourselves have an inevitable effect on how we move through the world, too: what we notice or fail to notice, what we obsess about and commit to memory, or what we look past or instantly forget. Our interpersonal relationships are all affected by story (which is why I tell so many in my books). Most powerful of all, though, is *how you are describing yourself to yourself.* That's both affected by mood and attitudes, and also shifts and shapes mood and attitude.

The story I want to tell is actually a legend. That means it is not quite true and also more than true. *Like so much that's happening in your mind.* The hero of this story is a young Jewish woman called Martha. She's the sister of the woman known in Christian scriptures as Mary/ Myriam, the sister of Martha and their brother, Lazarus.

Martha was the practical sister left to get on with all the many tasks of hospitality while Mary sat with their friend, Jesus, rather than helping when he visited their home. But the legend I am sharing comes from a later time in their lives, when they moved from the village of Bethany in Galilee to a village in Provence, in the south of France.

This is an area of France that I know quite well. It has a remarkable quality of light. It is beautiful now. It was beautiful then. It has also inspired many artists, especially Impressionists who succeeded through their art to shift what the viewer "sees" from something realistic— perhaps predictable or even formulaic—to something that represents their "impressions," plus the fleeting nature of what they are seeing.

That is relevant to us, too, as we rethink our "impressions," questioning their "reality" or inevitability, and notice how our feelings change as our mood and perspective also change. In other words, *nothing is static.* Life is not "still." It is dynamic. So are you. It's wonderful to capture a moment in paint or memory, but you cannot stay there no matter how you try. Your "impressions" move like clouds across the sky of your mind. Though what affects you most are your fundamental attitudes, whether these are healing or harming, fearful or calming, unkind or kind. Which takes us back to Martha.

How or why Martha and her sister and brother found their way from Galilee to Provence, I can't tell you. What I can tell you with confidence is that Martha's tough experiences of loss, grief, and displacement gave her a depth of character that few if any people have who haven't known suffering. This doesn't justify suffering. Nor should it persuade us to resign ourselves to it. But experience can teach us what suffering is, and that we can do everything in our power to relieve it in our own lives and in the lives of other people. That's what Martha was called to do when the village where they ended up was visited by a dragon that unsurprisingly terrified the villagers.

The villagers' first impulse was to slay the dragon. (Isn't that what heroes do—kill what endangers them?) Martha's way was different. First, she sprinkled the tail of the dragon with holy water. Then she tied her own silken belt around its middle. Did she speak soothing words to the dragon while she did this? Did she reassure the dragon that while it couldn't stay, she would not harm it? We can't know that for sure. What we do know is that Martha led the dragon out of the village, and *the dragon allowed itself to be led.*

Treating an unwelcome visitor (to our minds) with kindness as well as skill is a choice with limitless positive consequences. As with all legends, each of these characters is an archetype that resonates inside you and me. Each of us is Martha, the terrified villager, and the dragon. Each of us is also a listening, observing, discerning whole self, capable of choice except at the most extreme of times.

Martha's choices, and the delicacy with which she soothed the dragon, move me greatly and give me hope. My inner "Martha" is alive and well. (So is my inner contemplative Mary, and even my inner "Lazarus," who was raised from unconsciousness to consciousness, just as in "Once was blind, but now I see." That, though, is quite another story.)

What would change if you were to treat yourself with greater kindness? How

*would that change your experiences of suffering, your anxiety, your disrupted
moods and the anger and irritability, even despair, that can come with them?*

"I hate myself" is a cry of despair. It should never be ignored, any
more than "I hate my life" should be. Each is a cry from the soul—
whether you believe you have a soul or not. *How could you sprinkle holy
water onto the "tail" of your despair? How could you move your silken belt
(that keeps things secure) from one part of your body-mind to where it is most
needed?*

I can't provide you with answers. But you can. Viewing the big
story of your life with interest and compassion, seeing particular events
as not "stuck" but available to change, you grow into your maturity,
as well as your whole self. It's quite a shift that I am urging, but everything in this book supports my belief that it's possible. It's also quite a
shift to move forward a couple of thousand years from Martha's time
to ours, and from the insights of legend to the insights of a famous
contemporary playwright, Tennessee Williams. He certainly understood as you do how complex life can be, how unfairly demanding:
that it can cause us agonies as well as bring us contentment, amazement, and bliss. He knew as you do that to fulfill an intention to be
fully alive—even in the presence of dragons—requires trust, trust, and
more trust. And kindness and fortitude to sustain that.

In Williams's gorgeous words: "The world is violent and mercurial—
it will have its way with you. We are saved only by love—love for
each other and the love that we pour into the art we feel compelled to
share . . . We live in a perpetually burning building and what we must
save from it, all the time, is love."

These words from Tennessee Williams were not previously familiar
to me. They came to me in the last days of finishing this book. There

are many teachings on love in the book collection that spreads all over my house. There are many teachings also in my mind. Yet there's something so robust and rugged about the images that Williams evokes that it struck me as what I need. And you, too?

In our twenty-first-century threatened global world, we live not with dragons only—inside our minds or beyond them—but in a "perpetually burning building." It takes formidable courage to grow into all we can be. It takes stubbornness and grit to resist shrinking into superficiality or cynicism. In a world of constant communication, so little is said and so much wisdom is avoided.

Compliance with others' restricted views of who or what we are, or should be, is to be resisted. We need to lift our eyes up to a bigger vision of humankind and find ourselves there. A bigger view is what our world needs. It is certainly what we deserve.

We are not made to live fearfully.

What I long for you to feel within yourself is self-trust, even more than self-love. That's made the difference for me. Self-trust, hard-won, has taken me further into life, into my life with its inevitable contradictions. It has made me a less anxious person. It has transformed some, if not all, of my anxieties into more productive and creative actions, into Martha moments when I could treat myself with kindness rather than harshness.

Will I always be brought back to my child-self powerlessness when someone I dearly love is seriously threatened? Yes, probably. Will I continue to doubt my adequacy to do "enough," even when "enough" is way out of reach? Possibly. Will I still have to recognize some of my trauma scars through the dreams where I wake myself crying out? Yes. And yes.

In many other ways, however, I am freer with age and insight. My life has been unconventional in so many ways from my childhood onward. Creativity—using my imagination, instincts, curiosity, and drive to know more—has been and is a savior to me. So has my spiritual practice, which comes down to something as simple as regarding my life as part of a wondrous whole, a universe of infinite proportions that can never be understood in its entirety. In a far smaller, far more intimate way, you and I are also more than can be known in our entirety.

I like it, too, that Tennessee Williams, very far from a "perfect" human being, was remarkably creative. His perceptions on life—complex and robust—speak to me today as I write this. And speak to our times. This is not the creativity that you may believe belongs only to those making art or legends. It is the creativity that is as old as humankind, that is as varied as human nature, that is as natural as belonging and breathing. And loving.

Reducing anxiety, restoring trust, saving and savoring love: these are the lifelong gifts that you likely yearn for. *And can give yourself*— never to benefit yourself alone (that's not possible), but to play your part in bringing about a kinder, more awake, more fully alive world.

Throughout this book, I have offered starting, not finishing points. I will say again, you know yourself better than anyone else ever can, but you have been strenuously conditioned *not to see that fully*. Or to act on that self-knowledge. Then Anxiety with a capital "A" comes along to further limit the way you see yourself.

That tiny vignette about Martha, her silk scarf and her ability to turn a potentially violent act of shunning (the dragon) into an act of kindness and love, owes everything to the creative imagination of the legend-teller. It speaks, too, to your own legend-teller's mind, as much as it does to mine.

With inspiration and motivation on your side—remembering again that storytelling is the default position of your brain—you give yourself an opportunity to see your suffering differently: more compassionately, and certainly not as all that you are. You live in a crazy-anxious world. Your own courage and kindness have gotten you this far. Plus, you have unlimited inner resources to take you where you want to go.

To regard yourself more spaciously and generously, more *truthfully*, is just a step away. And the very next step is *to act differently*: with greater self-trust, and far more creatively.

Writer and famed psychiatrist Phil Stutz suggests that "the highest creative expression for a human being is to be able to create something in the face of adversity, and *the worse the adversity, the greater the opportunity* [my italics]." Why? How?

The "why" is because you and I are creatures of habit. Some (much) of our anxiety is habitual. Some (many) of our responses feel embedded because they are. This is not your "fault." Not at all. In fact, I notice at every in-person workshop I run how quickly people make a nest of their chair. Bags, a shawl, books—all saying, "Mine." Then, when I suggest that everyone change places after an hour, or a day, or yet again, there's frequently a reluctance to shift physically, to make a small gesture of "another beginning."

Our thinking goes the same way. We circle the nest. We land repeatedly where it's familiar. Even if it's desperately uncomfortable. Maybe, too, we are reluctant to risk hope. I understand that. *"Dare I try? Suppose my hopes are dashed—again?"* Yet, yet, yet, circling the same problems in the same way, on and on, *strengthens those problems*—and may consolidate your experiences of inadequacy. A catalyst is needed to bring about real change, strong enough to say, "Yes, I need to see myself differently. *My actions need to reflect that change.*" Can anxiety be such a motivator? Once it's uncomfortable enough, I believe it can.

The "how" gets more interesting. It sums up what I have named here as a whole-self perspective with a push from soul or spirit. This may be your unconscious positive drives, your instincts for healing. Stutz calls it *life force.* I'm happy with that. It's more than *will.* It's existential. And, thinking back to my earliest failed therapy, I realize that there was no life force conjured up between us, no palpable sense of moving forward, no summoning of strengths, no explicit, articulated encouragement to *live.* Just waiting. And waiting, however empathic, isn't enough. (Notable that a mental leap forward is so closely mirrored by the urging to move your body forward that's come everywhere in these pages.) But something else matters, too.

To make a big change in your thinking and attitudes, then translate that into effective action, *you need to embrace the possibility of change.* You need to open the door of your heart to the possibility of feeling more fully alive. *Trust what you have already survived.* Trust the courage you have stored up. Trust that only those of us who know fear, also know what it takes to meet it. Despite your loathing of it, anxiety will keep on colonizing you as long as you are not heading in a different direction. Fleeing the nest. Because you can. One short flight at a time.

Depression, too, will always color your thinking bleak. But your mind's power can *work for you*, not against you. Again and again, I have asserted in these pages that those of us who suffer anxiety will possess a powerful mind, a powerful imagination. How else could we conjure up all that might go wrong? Or replay so effectively all that has already gone wrong?

Dr. Stutz has pointed out that your inner world is so potent "it overwhelms [your] ability to see reality." That's true. Robbing you of confidence—and power—is one of anxiety's worst crimes. Shaking up your vision of *yourself* in passionate response is a profoundly creative act.

It can be life-changing. Or lifesaving. It can be an act of love.

Acknowledgments

I acknowledge the Gadigal people of the Eora Nation and those of the Larrakia Nation on whose lands this book was written. Also, the people of the Gomeroi Nation, including members of our own extended family. I pay my deepest respect to their Elders, past and present. Sovereignty on their lands has never been ceded.

Writing this book, I have been grateful for the wisdom of some quite exceptional writers. Most of what I have learned, however, is from the people whose suffering and courage I have witnessed firsthand, including those whose stories are glimpsed in these pages. I cannot name you but know that you are remembered always with gratitude and love.

I want to thank three friends: musician/composer Professor Kim Cunio, interfaith minister Rev. Hilary Star, and Zen Roshi Subhana Barzaghi, for years of standing close by spiritually. There are several writing and therapist friends who were kind enough to read or discuss early chapters and to share invaluable responses with me. They include Lisa Alther very particularly; Dr. Mark S. Burrows, Catherine Gilberd, Dr. Sally Gillespie, Dr. Jane Goodall, Dr. Margie Gottlieb, Dr. Richard Griffiths, Joyce Kornblatt, and Jane Moore.

What a pleasure it is to thank my St. Martin's Essentials publisher, Joel Fotinos, who brings to the vital collaboration between publisher and writer such warmth and unflagging encouragement—and an exceptional eye for what matters most. After seven books together, I could not be more grateful. At St. Martin's, I also want to thank Joel's excellent editorial assistant, Emily Anderson, whose enthusiasm for the publishing profession delights me and echoes my own; also Sophia Lauriello who, as senior publicist, is responsible for letting readers know the book exists (!). Sophia does that with skill, yes, plus a beautiful commitment to reaching readers. Austin Adams is key to the book's marketing success, and I am so happy to thank him, plus the many colleagues in marketing and sales whose names I don't yet know but on whom I most gratefully depend. My thanks are

279

also and always with my originating publishers, Allen & Unwin, and most particularly with Elizabeth Weiss, who, like Joel Fotinos, truly values making complex ideas wholeheartedly accessible.

My family are always in my heart. I want to mention with greatest gratitude my adult son and daughter, Gabriel and Kezia. Unlimited thanks to my older sister, Geraldine, who has known me always. I want to celebrate Madeleine, Charlie, Lux, and all the children in our world who deserve the finest legacy of joyful vitality and peace, both without and within.

Someone who deserves accolades as well as thanks is my husband, Dr. Paul Bauert. Discovering how eagerly the brain likes surprises (even startlement), and how the mind welcomes a horizon that's ever-expanding, I am more than ever thankful that "Happiness and Its Causes" led him from Darwin, NT, to Kyoto, Japan. And, for us both, to writing (and life) lessons without end.

Resources

A diagnosis can be helpful. Understanding your own experiences and discovering what combinations of inner and outer support work most effectively for you is the best help of all. Also, at different times, you may need more or different support. Reach for that as an act of self-love and self-care. There are seven types of identified anxiety disorders: generalized anxiety disorder, social anxiety disorder, panic disorder, separation anxiety disorder, phobias, selective mutism (an inability to speak in certain social situations), and anxiety "not otherwise specified." The Diagnostic and Statistical Manual of Psychiatric Disorders (DSM) is the official guide used in the US and elsewhere to diagnose psychological disorders.

Generalized anxiety disorder (GAD) involves "excessive" anxiety and worry that lasts for at least six months and is experienced on more days than it is not. (That's lots and lots and lots of us. Nonetheless, we worry alone and need to address it.) The person (you?) with GAD must find it difficult to control the worry, and it must be associated with at least three of six symptoms: 1) having difficulty concentrating or irritability, 2) restlessness or 3) feeling on edge, 4) being easily fatigued, 5) muscle tension, and 6) disturbed sleep.

Having established kinder, more self-supporting habits, focus now on what engages you and feeds your curiosity, what connects you most strongly to life, remembering that your greatest resources will always be human ones, both personal and professional, the stories they tell you, and the newly encouraging stories you tell yourself.

Two books to mention specifically: the first is Martha Manning's memoir, *Undercurrents*, where she briefly mentions the story of Martha and her transformative kindness to the dragon, retold in my final chapter. Finding that prompt by "chance" as I was near completing this book, I had a beautiful experience of synchronicity. The other book to mention is Judith Orloff's *Emotional Freedom*. This is one of many books on the emotional freedom technique (EFT), which involves tapping acupressure points while using self-accepting statements. It has been shown to be soothing for many people, in part because its message is one of whole-person acceptance. Readers may choose to explore this simple technique further in book form or online or with a psychologist or therapist.

Of my own books, those I believe will be most useful to you are *Choosing Happiness, Creative Journal Writing*, and *Intimacy & Solitude. Choosing Happiness* supports your interactions with other people, knowing that trustworthy relationships are vital for your well-being. *Creative Journal Writing* enhances insight and creativity, in every aspect of your life. *Intimacy & Solitude* clarifies how you build identity, what you "carry" into your connections with others, as well as what you bring into time alone—to make those experiences, too, solid and positive.

The following list includes some, not all, books mentioned here, and more besides. Avoiding absolutes, I may not "agree" with all of these authors' ideas; in fact, I probably don't. But sometimes an idea will stimulate us enough to explore further. That's what self-knowledge demands. And gives.

Botton de, Alain, and Armstrong, John. *Art as Therapy*

Botton de, Alain. *Status Anxiety*

Bowditch, Clare. *Your Own Kind of Girl*

Bregman, Rutger. *Humankind: A Hopeful History*

Doidge, Norman. *The Brain's Way of Healing: Remarkable Discoveries and Recoveries from the Frontiers of Neuroplasticity*

Frankl, Viktor. *Man's Search for Meaning*

Garcia, Hector, and Miralles, Francesc. *Ikigai: The Japanese Secret to a Long and Happy Life*; *The Ikigai Journey: A Practical Guide to Finding Happiness and Purpose the Japanese Way*

Genova, Lisa. *Remember: The Science of Memory and the Art of Forgetting.*

Gillies, Aaron. *How to Survive the End of the World (When It's in Your Own Head): An Anxiety Survival Guide*

Goldberg, Natalie. *The Great Failure: My Unexpected Path to Truth*

Grosz, Stephen. *The Examined Life: How We Lose and Find Ourselves*

Haig, Matt. *Notes on a Nervous Planet*

Hanh, Thich Nhat. *Fear: Essential Wisdom for Getting through the Storm; Peace Is Every Step: The Path of Mindfulness in Everyday Life*

Harper, Faith G. *Unf*ck Your Brain: Using Science to Get Over Anxiety, Depression, Anger, Freak-Outs, and Triggers*

Horowitz, Alexandra. *On Looking: A Walker's Guide to the Art of Observation*

Kabat-Zinn, Jon. *Wherever You Go, There You Are: Mindfulness Meditation in Everyday Life*

Kalanithi, Paul. *When Breath Becomes Air*

Lamott, Anne. *Bird by Bird: Some Instructions on Writing and Life*

Maté, Gabor, and Daniel. *The Myth of Normal: Trauma, Illness & Healing in a Toxic Culture*

May, Rollo. *The Meaning of Anxiety*

McKay, Matthew et al. *The Dialectical Behavior Therapy Skills Workbook: Practical DBT Exercises for Learning Mindfulness, Interpersonal Effectiveness, Emotional Regulation & Distress Tolerance*

Meurisse, Thibault. *Dopamine Detox: A Short Guide to Remove Distractions and Get Your Brain to Do Hard Things*

O'Donohue, John. *Divine Beauty: The Invisible Embrace*; *Anam Cara: Spiritual Wisdom from the Celtic World*

O'Rourke, Claire. *Together We Can: Everyday Australians Doing Amazing Things to Give our Planet a Future*

O'Rourke, Meghan. *The Invisible Kingdom: Reimagining Chronic Illness*

Popova, Maria. https://www.themarginalian.org/ (SD: Impossible to recommend this award-winning literary blog highly enough.)

Sherine, Ariane. *Talk Yourself Better: A Confused Person's Guide to Therapy, Counseling and Self-Help*

Smith, Gwendoline. *The Book of Overthinking: How to Stop the Cycle of Worry*

Solomon, Andrew. *The Noonday Demon: An Atlas of Depression*

Stutz, Phil, and Michels, Barry. *The Tools: 5 Tools to Help You Find Courage, Creativity, and Willpower*

Sweeney, Jon M., and Burrows, Mark S. *Meister Eckhart's Book of Secrets: Meditations on Letting Go and Finding True Freedom*

Thomas, Lewis. "*To Err is Human,*" in *The Medusa and the Snail: More Notes of a Biology Watcher*

Tuama Ó, Pádraig. *In the Shelter: Finding a Home in the World*; *Poetry Unbound: 50 Poems to Open Up Your World*

Vanderheide, Hannah. "There's Only One Reason We Should Be Talking About Jelena Dokic Right Now," *The Sydney Morning Herald*

Wolf, Maryanne. *Reader, Come Home: The Reading Brain in a Digital World*

Index

dopamine, 145–149, 169
 "training" the brain, 146
dreams / dreaming, 92, 108, 145, 235

eating disorders, 21, 35, 155, 157, 266
"eco-anxiety," 251–252, (throughout)
emergency measures, 5, 59–119. *See also* medication; safety net
emotional intelligence, 23, 105, 194
emotionally flooded / overwhelmed, 20–21, 37, 73, 100, 180, 188, 203, 233–234
emotions, (throughout)
empathy, 92, 136–139
Exposure Response Prevention (ERP) therapy, 204, 206. *See also* OCD

fear, 13, 18, 26, 40, 71, 85, 89, 110, 112–115, 124, 126, 153, 175, 191, 206, 256, 273
 effects on the body, 163, 267, 270
 fear memories, 5, 88, 111–112, 183–185, 238, 262
 fear of failure (not coping), 85, 100, 132, 137, 175, 186
 taking charge of fear, 86, 113, 115, 143–144, 152–153, 162, 168, 182, 188, 227, 232, 233–236, 259, 276

First Nations, 193, 251.
 See also racism
Frankl, Viktor Emil, 49–55

gender, questioning, 193, 250, 266
genes / genetics, 127–128, 152, 166, 187, 191
Gillies, Aaron, 47
glucocorticoids (and sleep), 125
grief, 18, 21, 39, 40, 51, 52, 67, 151–154, 186, 221, 254, 255–256, 262, 270

Hahn, Thich Nhat, 112–114, 259–260
Haig, Matt, 172, 173
Hankir, Ahmed, 161
Harper, Faith G., 36
"helpless," "hopeless" and (challenging them), 47, 60, 66, 84, 105, 107, 113, 147, 163, 241–242, 250, 261–264
help / self-help, 78–79, 189, (throughout)
hormones, 5, 15, 26, 59, 62, 76, 110, 117, 125, 130, 141, 146–148, 149

identity, (throughout)
Ikigai, 49, 244–245
illness, chronic and acute, 51, 126, 156, 171, 204, 236, 254, 262
 mental, 53–54, 99, 107, 163, 166, 173, 191, 193, 255
 terminal, 166

Inner Critic, 3, 47, 48, 53, 85, 103, 179, 223, 262
inner Rescuer, 151–154, 262, 263
insight, (throughout)
insomnia (sleep, sleeplessness), 15, 23, 53, 59, 68, 73, 97, 102, 111, 151, 178, 257, 281
 cortisol, 15, 62, 77, 126, 216
 dopamine, 147
International OCD Foundation (IOCDF), 206
irritability (and stress hormones), 15, 26, 68, 73–80, 82, 97, 167, 272, 281
 "anxious depression," 68–69
I-Thou connection, 162–163, 164

journal / journalling, 185, 198, 216, 219, 231–232, 233, 282
Jung, Carl (also Jungian therapy), 31, 92, 161

kindness (including to yourself), 32, 108, 109, 113, 153, 155, 156, 157, 158, 168, 179, 189, 249, 266

laughter (also joy), 2, 50, 96, 98, 101, 222, 248, 264, 266
logotherapy, 52, 54, 79

serotonin, 146, 204–205

sexism, 21, 153, 156, 158, 177, 201

Sherine, Ariane, 106

sleep. *See also* insomnia
cortisol, 216
dopamine, 148
need for, 77, 97, 102, 126, 151, 178, 216, 257

Smith, Gwendoline, 168–169

social anxiety, 21, 49, 74, 76, 130–131, 193, 230, 257, 263, 266, 281
children and adolescents, 130–131, 193, 196, 201

social media, 31, 162, 174–175, 193, 225

Solomon, Andrew, 107

status anxiety, 99, 160, 193–194, 266

stigma (of mental illness), 163

stress, (throughout)
hormones (*see* hormones)

stress audit, 79, 102

Stutz, Phil, 275

Styron, William, 241–242

suicidal ideation (also suicide), 50, 54, 60, 68, 104, 162, 164, 191, 193. *See also* despair

supraventricular tachycardia (SVT), 64

temperament, 128, 263

thinking (also insights) / thoughts, (throughout)

trauma, 18, 23, 26, 32, 39, 40, 51, 88, 126, 128, 141–142, 153, 161, 163, 170, 187, 191, 205, 238, 256, 263, 265, 273

Tuama O, Pádraig, 171, 268

vagal maneuvers, 65, 66–67

vagus nerve, 65

Vanderheide, Hannah, 157

venting (vent), 102, 217–220, 232

visualizations, positive, 13, 132–133, 224–230

"voices," inner, 47, 173

vulnerability, 3, 36, 60, 74, 75, 78, 124, 135, 138

wholeness, 30–31, 32, 39, 213

whole self (perspective and experience), 6, 8, 12, 18, 30–34, 37, 40, 41, 43, 67, 86, 94–96, 112, 114, 119, 134, 156, 158, 160, 164, 179, 182, 190, 212, 213, 230, 232, 241, 243, 244, 256, 271, 276

whole-self breathing, 67, 94–96

Williams, Tennessee, 272, 274

ABOUT THE AUTHOR

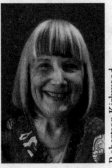

Robertson Kirkwood

STEPHANIE DOWRICK, PhD, DMin, has won international awards for three of her books: *Choosing Happiness, Creative Journal Writing,* and *Heaven on Earth.* A former leading publisher and psychotherapist, she is Australia's most original and successful personal and social development writer.

Her much-loved bestsellers also include *Intimacy & Solitude, Forgiveness & Other Acts of Love, The Universal Heart, Seeking the Sacred,* and *Everyday Kindness.* She has written fiction for adults and children, contributes widely to mainstream and social media, and is also known for her public speaking and workshop/retreat leadership in person and via Zoom, benefitting hundreds each year.

Dowrick was born in Aotearoa/New Zealand, spent sixteen years in Europe—mainly in the UK where she cofounded the Women's Press in London—and now splits her time between Sydney and Darwin.

Visit the author online at:
www.facebook.com/StephanieDowrick
www.stephaniedowrick.com